PRAISE FOR THE MINDBODY JOURNEY

'Thank you for an amazing and powerful Journey.'

'The MindBody Journey was one of the best things I've ever done'.

'The MindBody Journey is excellent. At this time in my life it has been the answer to a new beginning.'

'Loved it Jakkie. I'm a fan.'

'Thank you, I'm beginning to feel a new me!'

'I have finally discovered the reason behind my back pain.'

'I discovered my own fears and my will power to change anything I wanted.'

'I became self aware and had amazing insight into my blockages and what stopped me from going forward.'

'Jakkie is amazing and so good at explaining everything.'

'The MindBody Journey exceeded my expectations.'

'Thank you so much Jakkie. You have made such a difference to my life already and I am looking forward to being the new me!'

'I have gained so much and have a better understanding of myself and my course in life - Thank you.'

'How amazing it would be if this was taught in schools!'

'It was great to discover why my body was so out of balance and to be able to correct it'.

'Jakkie has bought a new wisdom and way of being into my life.'

'I gained an understanding of myself. How to believe in myself, understanding the reasons behind my physical conditions and I gained valuable tools on how to change my view of myself.'

'Thank you for all your help & guidance over the past year, I wish I had met you sooner. Your MindBody Journey has changed my life, and my mum's, and your energy and outlook is one to be forever admired.'

'I gained a greater understanding of myself and my thoughts and putting this into practice. I loved Jakkie. She was incredibly giving, supportive, extremely knowledgeable. An Inspiration.'

'Completing the MindBody Journey has completely changed my health, body and posture, relationships, happiness and my way of thinking and behaving. Thank you Jakkie for the opportunity to do this.'

'I finally found myself.'

**Feedback from people who completed
The MindBody Journey with Jakkie.**

Your MindBody Journey

Change your mind, heal your body, transform your life

JAKKIE TALMAGE

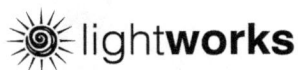

☀ light**works**

Your MindBody Journey

change your mind, heal your body,
reshape your life

JANICE TALMAGE

lightworks

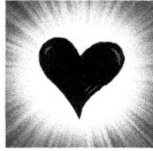

'I do not fix my problems.
I fix my thinking.
Then problems fix themselves'.

Louise Hay

'Intelligence is present everywhere
in our bodies...our own innate intelligence
is far superior to any we can try to
substitute from the outside'.

Deepak Chopra

To all my clients,
for without you and your
bravery to transform your lives,
this book would not exist

CONTENTS

A NOTE FROM THE AUTHOR

One day I was sitting in a seafront café in Sussex England, having a nice cup of tea with a friend, listening to her complain about how painful her left shoulder was.

She's a massage therapist, and because I had worked as a sports therapist for many years, I know just how exhausting it can be treating a lot of bodies in one day. So I nodded in an empathetic way that said 'I know how you feel'.

And then I asked her the all important question: 'Why?'

She pursed her lips a little and narrowed her eyes as if to say 'do we have to go there?', but I persisted like only good friends can.

'Why do you think your arm and shoulder is so painful?'

Her face told me she wanted to say something like, 'because I've been doing eight bloody massages a day, why do you think it's so painful?'. But she knew that I know about the MindBody connection, that the mind and body are not separate and that all our aches, pains and symptoms can nearly always be traced back to the mind.

So I asked her again, 'Why is it REALLY hurting? What is your shoulder REALLY saying to you', and once she realised that resistance was futile, she relaxed into the conversation, which went something like this:

Me, "So what is the 'feeling' behind your hurty shoulder?'

Her, 'Well it feels achey, tired, exhausted even!'

Me, 'What are the feelings behind the achey, tired exhausted feeling?'

Her, 'It feels angry.'

Me, 'Whats behind the anger?'

Her, 'RESENTMENT!'

That word flew out of her mouth with such a fierce spit, I almost had to duck!

Me, 'Why are you resentful?'

Her, 'Because every time I get a client on the couch I wish it was ME. I am soooo in need of pampering and being given to, but all I seem to do is give, give, give, I feel sucked dry of energy. I want to be the one that receives for a change. I've had enough!'

And as the word 'enough' flew out of her mouth she thrust her left palm towards me to indicate 'stop', sending a spasm of pain through her shoulder and then she burst into tears.

From a MindBody perspective, all of this made perfect sense. The left side of her body represents her feminine needs and qualities such as nurture, passivity and a desire to receive. The arms represent the world of 'doing'---and she was clearly doing too much doing---while the shoulder usually represents the things in life we are carrying. Her body was yelling 'enough, enough, enough' and her desire to thrust out her arm and make it all stop had created a build up of unexpressed, angry emotion that was trapped in her left shoulder.

Having MindBody insights like this is all well and good, but if you don't act on this knowledge, then the physical problem will persist. It wasn't until she was able to acknowledge the resentment she was feeling, because of all the hard work and caring for others she was doing, and take some action to get her own needs met, that the problem started to shift.

The next time we met a few months later in the same café, her shoulder pain had completely disappeared and she spent the whole afternoon telling me how much happier she was, now she was saying 'no' more and giving more time for herself and doing things she loved.

Over the years I've helped many women and men to use the MindBody connection as a vehicle to help them change their lives for the better, often in profound and dramatic ways. Yet this brief, informal exchange with a dear friend reminds me of how easy it can be to make changes in our lives, when we learn to trust our inner knowing.

And so this book has been written with that spirit of friendship and simplicity in mind, for people like you, who are ready to share in the ancient wisdom of the MindBody connection.

With Blessings
Jakkie Talmage
Sydney, Australia, January 2016

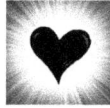

PART ONE: Your Mind

Your MindBody Journey is structured in three distinct parts, which focus on thinking (your mind); doing (your body) and being (your soul).

In Part One of the book there's lots of useful information that's designed to prepare you mentally for your journey of discovery. In this section you'll learn about the MindBody connection and find out how the thoughts you think are having a direct impact on both your body and your life.

The key to understanding how your thoughts and words influence your health and wellbeing, is through the mastery of your own MindBody language.

By learning to read the messages from your unconscious mind, that are hidden in your MindBody, you will prepare yourself to take the journey of a lifetime to health, happiness and success.

CHAPTER ONE

Your MindBody Journey

Welcome to Your MindBody Journey.

This book is for you and about you. It is designed to help you embark on your own personal journey to discover the remarkable connections between your mind, your body and your life. Throughout Your MindBody Journey, you'll uncover the blocks that have been preventing you from reaching your full potential, having full health and following your life purpose.

Over the years I've worked with hundreds of clients, each facing their own unique set of challenges, and I've discovered we all have one thing in common---the biggest barrier that stops us from reaching our fullest potential, in every area of our life, is our own minds.

Of course you may already know this at some level, but have you ever noticed that knowing something doesn't always make a difference?

You may know how to ride a bike, for example, but you can't teach a child to ride a bike by just telling her how to do it or giving her a book to read. Yes you can guide your child and give her advice and help her balance on her bike, but ultimately she has to learn how to ride the bike with her own body---she has to 'embody' the knowledge.

This is how Your MindBody Journey works.

What's Stopping You?

I know from my own experience of taking people on this voyage of personal discovery, that this book will show you how to embody each of the personal discoveries you make in a way that can make a profound difference in your life.

You'll do this by tapping into the power of a very simple MindBody secret.

You see, the reason you may struggle to overcome the mental blocks that prevent you from living the life you want to live, is that you can't see these blocks. And the reason you can't see them is because they're hidden from view, deep in your unconscious mind.

You probably know this already, because if you could see these mental blocks then you know you would do something about them.

Of course sometimes it's easier to blame external factors for the fact that we're not fully living the life we want to live. We point the finger at our parents, our partners, our education, our luck, our past decisions, our circumstances and so on.

And of course we may be right about all of these external factors, but being right about things that are outside of our control, rarely makes a difference. What does make a difference is looking inwards and uncovering the personal blocks that prevent us from living a life we love no matter what our circumstances. And when we do this, when we change what's happening inside, then our external circumstances tend to change anyway, just like magic!

The MindBody Secret

One way to uncover these blocks is by exploring your Mind-Body connection.

As you may be aware, your thoughts, beliefs and memories don't just live in your head, they are held in every nerve and cell in your body. You know this because when you remember a happy memory you don't just see it in your mind's eye, you feel it throughout your body. This is your MindBody in action.

Once you realise that every positive and negative thought you ever had is held in your MindBody, you can use this knowledge to uncover all the unconscious blocks that are holding you back from living a life you love and deserve.

The secret to uncovering these mental blocks is simple---the mental blocks that are holding you back are not just hidden in your unconscious mind, but they are also hidden throughout your body. They are 'embodied'.

This is the MindBody secret.

So, if you are ready to discover the mental blocks that are preventing you from living the life you want to live, and the health you were born to have, then you need look no further than your own body.

Because the thoughts you think, not only give you the life you live, but also give you the body you embody.

You Can Create The Life You Want

If you want to change your life, then you need to change your thoughts, and the way to start that journey is by asking your body which thoughts and beliefs are no longer working for you.

This is the journey that this book will take you on. With the help of a series of thought experiments, physical exercises and powerful visualisations, you are about to embark on your own personal MindBody journey to a healthier, happier, more successful future.

Sound too good to be true? Well, it's all up to you!

You have the power to create a life you want, or a life you don't want. You create everything in your life. That's how powerful you are. So instead of creating poor health, unhealthy relationships, dissatisfaction in your work and home life, why not create the opposite? You can experience peace and happiness in every moment, but most of us are lucky if we even get passing glimpses of this elevated state of being every now and then.

So what stops you from feeling peace and happiness all of the time? This is what you will discover on Your MindBody Journey. Once you uncover and remove the hidden blocks that prevent you from being peaceful and happy in each and every moment, then you will have discovered your personal heaven on earth.

The Tale Of The Crying Monk

I first became aware of the power of the MindBody connection in 1996 when I was working as a massage therapist. I was living in Australia at the time and working in a Yoga Centre in Sydney.

A woman came to the centre asking for a massage, so I booked her in for an hour-long treatment. She was a Buddhist monk who lived in a nearby ashram and although she was young, she was as tiny and frail as a woman three times her age.

She was also very quietly spoken and didn't say a word other than to tell me that her mother had paid for her treatment, as she couldn't afford to pay for it herself. She complained of a bad back and tiredness.

As soon as I started the massage she began to cry. I was worried I was hurting her frail body, but she assured me I wasn't and asked me to continue. For the whole hour she cried big, loud sobs. After the treatment she got up, thanked me, dressed and went home.

I didn't expect to see her again. I assumed she wouldn't come back if my treatment was so awful that it made her cry like a baby! But she was back the next week and the week after that and every time she came, the same thing happened. She would sob and sob for a whole hour, then get dressed and leave.

I learnt not to ask questions and to accept that this is what she needed to do. On her 18th session with me an amazing thing happened---she didn't cry! Her muscles felt soft and she was no longer rigid. When she got off the couch she said, 'Thank you, I am now healed'.

After that session I never saw her again. I did however see her face in the local newspaper a year later and discovered she had cured herself of cancer and was now helping others to heal!

Looking back I realise those treatments were a key part of her recovery. Whatever mental blocks she had been holding onto in her body had been released and she was now free from her past suffering and creating a future she loved and deserved.

Now that I am an experienced MindBody practitioner, I know it doesn't need to take 18 massages to uncover and release the blocks that are holding you back.

You don't have to suffer, get ill, shout, scream or cry for a month to become well (unless of course you believe you do!) All you have to do to be free from anything that doesn't work for you in your life---be it your relationships, your poor health, your lack of financial security, your depression---is change the programming and belief systems that are locked in your MindBody. It is as simple as that.

Time For A Personal Upgrade?

To do this we first need to understand what makes us tick.

So, why is it that we keep repeating the same health issues, the same problematic relationships, the same patterns in our finances? The answers lie in our unconscious programming.

We spend most of our lives operating through our unconscious programming, largely unaware of the thoughts and beliefs that are shaping our lives. Our unconscious mind is far more powerful than our conscious mind.

According to biologist, Dr Bruce Lipton, our subconscious mind is a million times more powerful than our conscious mind, and we spend 95 percent of our lives operating through unconscious programming that most of us are not aware of.

Now, this is the scary bit! Our life is being run by hidden thoughts and beliefs that are largely invisible and unknown to us. This unconscious programming is usually set up during our childhood and even the thoughts and emotions of our mother while we were in her womb.

Dr Lipton says we download the majority of this unconscious programming between the ages of 0-6 years old, mostly from our parents and the culture we're born into. All of our early experiences are directly downloaded into our subconscious, then we spend the rest of our lives being driven by this programming, until such time as a new program or pattern is set up.

Every nerve, cell and fibre in our body follows orders from our unconscious mind.

Bruce discovered that fewer than five percent of us are born with faulty genes, which means that the vast majority of disease that we suffer is caused by our lifestyles, which includes the actions we take, the thoughts we believe and the stress we create for ourselves.

The neural pathways in our brains are like superhighways packed with nerve cells constantly sending instructions to the rest of our body, and once we have programmed ourselves to do a certain task, in a certain way, we will keep on doing it until we are programmed to do things differently.

In this respect we are very much like a computer. The way a computer works and responds depends on what software program has been installed. If the computer operator is using outdated software, the operator will probably blame the computer when things don't go right, or the system's too slow, or it breaks down.

If however the computer is upgraded with new software and programming, then things go smoothly and everything works perfectly. It is up to you to recognise when the old way of doing things, your old programming doesn't work anymore and when the time has come for you to give yourself a personal upgrade!

Where Did Your Beliefs Come From?

The irony is that because we think things 'happen to us' we believe our 'luck' is a matter of fate, or just the way things are. We say things like 'I've always been unlucky in love' or 'I always fail' or 'my bad health runs in the family', and we believe what we are saying is true.

And because we believe these thoughts to be true---and because human beings love to be right---then the thoughts we think keep coming true. The things we believe keep happening to us, locking us into a vicious circle of negative programming. Yet when we understand that we unconsciously set up beliefs like 'I'm always unlucky in love' or 'I always fail', then we can let go of those beliefs and replace them with new thoughts and beliefs that help us create the life we want to live.

In many cases it is a simple incident that happened in our childhood (or even in adulthood) which set up our recurring thoughts and belief systems. It may be an incident we've forgotten about, but our unconscious mind is still holding onto. And so this unconscious memory runs our lives, always present in the background, secretly guiding us in our thoughts and our actions.

This emotional baggage has a tendency to follow us around wherever we go, tripping us up, holding us back and sabotaging our search for happiness and success. Because these belief systems feel so true to us, because we keep re-enforcing these beliefs with our thoughts, feelings and actions, it can sometimes be a struggle for us to change.

But it is possible with a bit of awareness, a lot of practice and a big dollop of patience.

Everyone's Personal Story Is Unique

Maybe a playground bully created a belief within us that we are unlovable. Perhaps a parent who wanted us to do well in our exams and got disappointed when we didn't perform, created a belief system within us that we'll never be good enough. It could be a mother or father who left the family unit who created a belief system that somehow we were to blame and so we believe we are never to be trusted.

When we broke a leg playing on the school sports field and had to be rushed to hospital, we created a belief system that we are accident prone. When we were discouraged from doing what we love, and encouraged to do what our parents and teachers thought was best for us instead, we created a belief system that others know better and that we shouldn't listen to our heart.

When we were told that money is scarce and we must watch every penny or we will always be poor, we created a belief system of lack and scarcity. When we were told that we must work hard and long hours to ever be a success, we began to believe that digging ourselves into an early grave and working to excess is the only way to achieve.

As human beings, we are designed to learn from our mistakes, but sometimes this can hinder us more than helps us. The unconscious, repetitive, negative thoughts we think about ourselves and our lives on a daily basis, are usually beliefs we made up to protect us from pain in the past. By holding onto these past-based thoughts in the present moment, we prevent ourselves from experiencing more pleasure and happiness in the future.

Your Biography Is Your Biology

Not only do our thoughts and belief system create the life we live, but they also show up physically in our body. This is where the clues are. Each part of your body has a story to tell and expresses this story in its own MindBody language.

Our body reflects all the experiences and events we've ever had in our lives so far. Because the thoughts we think, have not only given us the life we have lived, but also the body we have embodied.

This means that our past is evident in our posture, our body shape, the way we speak, the way we move, the way we function and the way we operate. We are the sum total of everything that has happened to us. This includes the programming we inherited from our parents, our schooling, our hurts and upsets, our personal resentments and all the negative and positive experiences we've had so far.

We adopt certain habits, which help to keep us safe in life, to protect our vulnerabilities and our perceived inadequacies. This is our programming and sometimes it doesn't serve us in a positive way. If an unresolved emotion or trauma has not been released, then it remains in our body as an energy block and then eventually results in dis-ease. We'll cover what our energy is in chapter 3.

The most common energy blocks are shaped by the negative attitudes or fear based thoughts that we carry around with us. The thoughts we keep thinking affect our nervous system, our endocrine system and eventually our immune system. Put simply, a happy mind is a healthy body and an unhappy mind is an unhealthy body.

Every thought you have is communicating to your body, producing either stress responses or healing responses, switching your genes on or off. In order to heal yourself and to feel a sense of peace, happiness and wellbeing, all you have to do is throw out your old attitudes and destructive, negative thought patterns.

Such thoughts start in our mind, yet they quickly manifest in your body as stiff shoulders, digestive disorders, headaches, back aches and panic attacks and can eventually turn into more serious illnesses like cancer and heart disease.

It's All In Your DNA

We were once led to believe that it was our DNA, passed down from our ancestors, that was responsible for our health and programming. If our mother, father or grandparents had a particular disease or disorder, then it was inevitable that we would be prone to the same illnesses. However more recent studies have shown that it is the beliefs that are passed down to us from our ancestors, which shape our genetic makeup.

Experiments undertaken by the Institute of HealthMath have revealed the powerful impact our thoughts can have on our DNA.

When volunteers were asked to focus on joy, love, gratitude and appreciation their DNA strands became relaxed and started to unwind. When the volunteers focused on thoughts of fear, hate, anger, guilt, frustration or any other destructive emotion, the DNA strands tightened and became shorter, and some genes even switched off altogether.

So we literally 'unwind' when we become relaxed and get 'wound up' when we are stressed. What researchers are now finding is that our minds are so powerful that they can even change our genetic blueprint!

So consider this. Your body is constantly changing and evolving. Seven million of your red blood cells die and reform every second. Every four days you will grow a new stomach lining, to prevent it from digesting itself! Your skin regenerates every seven days. Every seven years your bones are fully rebuilt. Your mind and your beliefs will reshape your cells and your bones. If you keep holding onto the same attitudes and thoughts, then you will keep recreating the same body. If you change the way you think and see the world, you will transform and create a totally new body.

You Have The Power To Transform Your Life

The simple premise of Your MindBody Journey is that by changing your thoughts you can heal your body and transform your life. The first step on this journey is self-awareness.

Tapping Into Your Inner Wisdom

In my experience, once we remove the fear, then all the other excuses tend to disappear! Remember, fears are not real, they are just beliefs you made up to keep you safe.

It is said that F.E.A.R is the acronym for False Evidence Appearing Real.

If you want to find answers that will take you beyond these false fears, then all you need to do is tap into your inner wisdom. All the answers are already there within you. Your body is constantly talking to you. When you have an ache or pain, a bruise or even have an accident, it is your unconscious mind communicating with you.

The problem is that most of the time we don't or won't listen to the inner wisdom of our bodies. We would rather let someone or something else 'fix it', to take away the pain and discomfort as quickly as possible, so we can get on with our lives.

Yes we can fix things temporarily, but if we don't address the underlying issue, the root cause, then the problem will just keep coming back and even get worse!

We're often so busy rushing around attempting to create the illusion that we 'have it all' that we forget the single most important relationship we have---our relationships with ourselves and our own bodies.

It doesn't matter whether you like the look, shape, feel, or how it behaves, your body is your most important friend. If you see your body as an enemy rather than your faithful friend and servant, then you will never be healthy, happy and at peace.

Your body operates 24 hours a day, every day of every week, working relentlessly to keep you healthy so you can enjoy your life. Yet have you ever noticed how quick we are to get upset with our body when it breaks down, and how slow we are to thank it when we are in good health?

Preparing For Your Journey

Once we realise that we are the one's who create our body's poor health, we would not be so quick to criticise our body and we would do everything we could to serve our body, like it serves us. How much time do you spend listening to your body? Not much? How often do you act accordingly to change what you need to change? Not often?

All that is about to change. All your answers are already within you, it's time to for you to start accessing them. It's time to stop, listen and value yourself enough to hear what is really going on for you and for your truth to emerge. Being honest about what's really going on and taking responsibility for your own pain, be it emotional or physical, is a brave step to take! But what we resist, persists. You owe it to yourself and your future happiness to find your answers.

It is now time to listen.

In this book, you will take yourself on a MindBody Journey of self discovery that will change your relationship with your body and change your life in the process!

As you journey deeper and deeper you will uncover hidden messages in every part of your body. You will learn to listen to your intuition and the voice of wisdom within you. There are written questions for you to answer, physical exercises for you to experiment with and a series of meditations to prompt and guide you, every step of the way. You'll also read stories about other people who have already been on this journey, as I share their experiences with you.

You can take as little or as much time with this book as you like. You might want to read it through before you do the exercises, or even read it and NOT do the exercises. Whatever you feel you are ready to do. However if you really want to discover and release your own programming and unconscious patterns to fully change your health and life for the better, then I suggest, with intention, you make time and find a quiet space to do the practices fully.

Once you commit to your journey, try and resist the temptation to skip any of the exercises, because if you do you won't complete all the pieces of your jigsaw puzzle. You can do the exercises alone or share the journey with a friend who is also committed to transforming their life. The choice is yours.

Are you ready? Then lets begin!

KEY LESSONS FROM CHAPTER ONE

- **The thoughts you think have given you the life you live and the body you've embodied**

- **Your thoughts and beliefs are programmed in your unconscious mind and hidden from your view**

- **Learning to listen to your body is the key to uncovering these unconscious thoughts**

- **Changing your thoughts and beliefs will change your body and change your life**

CHAPTER TWO

Your MindBody Connection

Here is a simple explanation of how your MindBody connection works and plays out in your life. Your mind is directly linked to your nervous system and your nervous system is directly linked to your body, therefore every thought you have creates a reaction within your body.

Put another way, the thoughts that you think create the body you embody.

Here's a little thought experiment you can do to experience this MindBody process in action.

Imagine a big yellow lemon. Imagine you are holding it, feeling the skin of the lemon in your hands, smelling it's lemony flavours with your nose. Now imagine cutting that lemon into wedges with a knife. Notice the little spurts of citrus squirting onto your skin as you picture this. Think about the sound the knife makes as your cut through the yellow fruit. See if you can conjure up the bitter-sweet tang of the citric acid in the air.

Now imagine you are picking up a big wedge of lemon lifting it up to your mouth. Stick out your tongue and give the lemon a couple of cautious licks and the pretend to bite into the fleshy insides and taste the sharp, bitterness of the lemon's juices as they make your taste buds tingle.

Now, if you are really good at imagining and visualising things, then at least some of this exercise would have felt real for you. Maybe you noticed your taste buds spurting at the bitter taste of the imaginary lemon? Maybe it was the smell or the touch or even the sounds of the lemon that seemed real?

Whatever your experience, if your body and sensory system reacted to the thought of putting that imaginary lemon in your mouth, then this was your MindBody connection in action.

You Think And Feel With Your Whole Body

Put simply, the MindBody connection means that when you think of something your body reacts, because your mind and body aren't separate, they are connected as a single, unified system we call the MindBody.

So, you think of a food you love and your mouth starts to water. You think about an exam you have to take or an important meeting or interview and you get butterflies in your stomach. Even thinking of something simple like walking into a freezer can make you start to shiver.

So when you have fearful thoughts, then your body's automatic defence mechanisms kick in---your heart rate quickens, your breathing gets faster and your palms get sweaty. This is all automatic and is a good indication that your fight, flight and freeze hormones have kicked in.

If you repeatedly think anxious or negative thoughts over a period of time, then your nervous system will be in overdrive, depleting your immune system and resulting in energy blocks. Over time these blocks could manifest into pain, headaches, tight muscles, bad posture or malfunction in your organs and glands, resulting in sometimes more serious illnesses.

These observations aren't designed to scare you or to perpetuate your fearful thoughts, but to help empower you with the knowledge that YOU have the ability to create a healthy, happy, successful life. Because the thoughts you think everyday, create the body you embody and the life you keep living, each and every day.

Fight, Flight Or Freeze?

As you may be aware, human beings are conditioned to respond to stress in one of three ways, known simply as fight, flight or freeze. These evolved responses, that were once a matter of life or death, are linked to specific hormones that we still generate even though we now live in a much safer world than our ancestors did.

Our body is brilliantly designed, so that when we are in danger our HPA (hypothalamus, Pituitary and Adrenal) are instantly activated to prepare our body for action. Our adrenal cortex automatically releases adrenalin and cortisone into our body to help us deal with the danger. The thyroid gland automatically stimulates our metabolism and sends more oxygenated blood to our larger muscles and organs.

Unlike our ancestors, we are not constantly fleeing from the imminent threat of a sabre-toothed tiger or other life-threatening situations, but because our minds still respond to everyday stresses with fear-based thoughts, our bodies still believe we are in danger.

So what triggers your personal stress responses?

Is it traffic? Work deadlines? The daily barrage of calls, texts and social media alerts? The inbox full of emails? Your family responsibilities? Your finances? The media? Your career? Your social life? Your love life?

Whatever causes you stress, the chances are that your life is not threatened, but your body may be thinking you are in constant danger because of the stress messages your brain keeps sending it. And there is only so much stress that you can take before your body will start to show signs of distress and fatigue.

Learning To Love Your Thoughts

Scientists have found that mental and emotional stress reduces the levels of growth hormones (proteins that help the body to heal) at wound sites. So our body takes longer to heal when we are stressed. When our HPA is habitually activated, then it is likely that disease is imminent. Your body cannot heal itself as effectively if it is constantly responding to stress.

Every conscious and unconscious thought you have influences millions of atoms, molecules and cells throughout your body. Every thought you think has a corresponding vibrational frequency, ranging from high vibrations like love and low vibrations like fear, to all the emotional vibrations in between.

Research tells us that the simple act of consciously generating loving thoughts activates an immune response in our bodies. Yet most of us spend more time having unconscious, fear-based thoughts that pump us full of stress hormones.

All human beings have their own unique way of responding to stress and it is always a variation of the fight, flight or freeze response. As you start to become aware of your own Mind-Body connection, you will begin to notice different aspects of your personal programming.

Exercise #1:
Discover Your Personal Stress Response

Here's a simple exercise to help you consider how you respond to stress. It's a simple first step for you to take on Your MindBody Journey towards greater self-awareness.

If you think about the times in your life when you've faced stressful situations, what do you remember about how you responded? Pick an incident that you're happy to remember, not one that is too traumatic or painful. It could be a recent situation or any other time in your life.

Close your eyes and think back to that moment. Remember what you could see and hear around you, remember how you felt. Really tune into the feelings in your body and see if your can remember what your first instinct was? Was it a fight, flight or freeze response?

Notice what's going on in your body---your heart rate, your muscles, your jaw, your breathing.

If you are a fighter, you may have noticed an anger response during this exercise. Do you feel like you need to constantly fight battles to solve the problems you face?

If you are more of a 'flighter' than a 'fighter', you may have noticed you leg muscles twitching, priming yourself for flight. Do you prefer to walk away from confrontation and conflict other than facing problems head on?

If you are a freezer, you may have noticed yourself holding your breath or avoiding reliving the memory. Do you generally feel stuck when you are stressed, become paralysed or go into denial about the issues you pretend that don't exist?

Every person I've ever worked with has had a tendency towards one of these three automatic stress responses and has been unconsciously acting and reacting in this way, in times of stress, throughout their lives.

You may think you are mix of all three and you're probably right, but if you really think about it there'll be one response that you tend to favour. The MindBody impact of our favoured stress response is so powerful that it shows up in subtle ways in our body language. What did you notice about your body in that exercise.

Which is your preferred response, fight, flight or freeze?

What Your Body Language Can Tell You

If you are a **fight person**, for example, then you may clench your fists, clench your jaw or feel your breathing quicken when you are in stress. If you are stuck in the fight response, physical conditions can occur such as muscular aches and pains, hypertension, immune disorders and thyroid conditions.

If you are a **flight person** on the other hand, then you may unconsciously move your torso and feet away from a person or situation you dislike, ready to flee. Physical symptoms of someone severely locked in the flight response are burn out, hyperactivity, fibromyalgia and rheumatoid arthritis. If you are a flight person, next time you are at a meeting, or a gathering that you don't particularly want to be at, check the position of your feet. There is a good chance they're facing the exit ready for a quick escape!

If you are a **freeze person**, you may hold your breath, or cross your arms over your chest or close your eyes for protection. If you find you get stuck and unable to resolve ongoing issues and your foot is firmly on the brake, then you are possibly stuck in the freeze response. Physical conditions can manifest within the body and these include, low blood pressure, tiredness, depression, ME and water retention.

The Tale Of Two Stress Heads

Our stress responses can show up in unexpected ways. When my partner and I are running behind schedule our different stress responses can sometimes clash, because I tend to rush and he tends to slow down. This is because I am a flight person and he is a freeze person.

If we're not mindful of our programming, we sometimes find that my rushing can make him stressed so he goes even slower and his slowness can stress me out and make me rush more frantically. The more I rush the more he slows down and the more he goes too slowly the more I go too quickly. Eventually we become like a comical human version of a very annoyed hare and a very grumpy tortoise, with the result that we end up getting nowhere.

Of course we're not doing this deliberately to annoy each other, even though it can feel like it at the time, it's just our unconscious programming running the show. Once I've stopped trying to hurry him up and he's stopped trying to slow me down, we get to where we're heading and then have a good laugh at ourselves later (sometimes much, much later!).

So what about you? Are you a fight, flight or freeze person? Taking a little time to consider this simple question is a great way for you to start developing the self-awareness you will need to make the most of Your MindBody Journey.

If you find you can't work it out for yourself, or just want a second opinion, then it's a good idea to ask your family, friends or colleagues because if you haven't noticed how you react to the stress and challenges of life, they probably have!

KEY LESSONS FROM CHAPTER TWO

* Your body responds to whatever your mind is thinking, this is the MindBody connection

* All human beings have either a fight, flight or freeze response to stress

* Identifying your own personal stress response is the first step in developing your awareness of your Mind-Body connection

CHAPTER THREE

Getting To Know Your MindBody

Before you go on any journey it's a good idea to find out about the place you are visiting by looking at a map or reading a guide book.

This chapter is designed to give you the information you need to get more acquainted with your MindBody as you prepare to take the first steps on your own personal journey of discovery.

You'll learn some handy new phrases, find out about the places of interest you are going to visit and learn about the characteristics of the different regions of your body.

For example, if I told you that you have four main body centres, would you know what they are or where to find them? They are called your moving centre, your being centre, your doing centre and your control centre. Take a moment to see if you instinctively know where these centres are located in your body. We'll see how well you did in a moment!

Exercise #2:
Learning To Act With Confidence

First, do you remember in Chapter One we discussed how the thoughts you think, give you the body you embody and the life you live? Well we're going to take a look at an example of how your thoughts can shape your life. In the workshops I run, we do an exercise and you can try this now if you want to.

You'll need to stand up and have a little space to walk around. Then imagine what type of posture a person who thinks confident thoughts, feels confident feelings and acts in a confident way would have. How would they stand and hold themselves? Now walk around exaggerating the posture of someone who thinks, feels and acts in a confident manner.

When you've got a good feel for that character stop and give your body a good shake. Now do the opposite. Picture the posture of a person who isn't confident. Imagine how that type of person would hold themselves. Now walk around again exaggerating the posture of someone who thinks unconfident thoughts, feels unconfident feelings and acts in an unconfident manner.

Again stop and shake yourself down before taking a moment to reflect on the exercises. What did you notice by doing this? Did you notice that you felt different in each posture? Which way of holding yourself was closest to your normal posture---the confident character or the unconfident? And most importantly, what do you think comes first, the thoughts, the feelings or the posture?

In my experience, the magical thing about the MindBody connection is that when we start to change the way we hold our body, it can change the way we think and feel too.

And it's not just thoughts or feelings about how confident we are, that manifest in our body. Every thought and feeling we have is reflected in our body and different types of emotions and psychological blocks can show up in particular parts of our body, such as the four body centres.

So let's see how good your instinct was when you tried to guess where your four body centres are located.

Your Body Centres

Your Moving Centre is the area of your body between your hips and the ground. It includes your hips, your legs and your feet. Your feet indicate how grounded you are and how strong and stable you are when it comes to standing on your own two feet. Your ankles and knees represent your flexibility to change. Your legs represent your direction in life. Your hips represent support and stability, your foundation and security. Any issues in this centre, or messages from this part of your body, are probably about your direction or standing in life.

Your Being Centre is your torso and includes your chest, your tummy and your spine. This front part of your being centre represents how you are "being" out there in your everyday life. Your chest is where you feel a sense of aliveness. It is your feeling self, where you hold your feelings of love and pain. Its also home to your lungs which control your breath, your life force and your 'pranayama' (a Sanskrit word to describe the strength of your life force). Then there's your tummy, which is where you experience your gut feelings, your intuitive self. It holds your self esteem, your will power and the way you express your emotions.

Your being centre also incorporates your back, spine and central nervous system. Your spine is your life support. It is the backbone of your life and represents your ability to take responsibility for yourself. It is your own personal support network and relates to your core strength, your will and your personal power. Most of all it represents your ability to support yourself in life.

Your Doing Centre is your arms and shoulders. It connects with your torso and is a "channel" through which you express what's happening in your being centre. Your arms and shoulders express the things that you do in your life and how you do them. They express your love, your creativity and your personal needs and wants. Your doing centre expresses your 'being' through physical action.

Your right arm is representative of your masculine side, your giving self. It's about being assertive and active. It's your doing energy. Your left arm is representative of your feminine self, it's about being passive, intuitive and receiving. It's your being energy. Your shoulders connect your arms and channel your being energy into doing energy. They can also be used as a form of protection, for example when they hunch up around your neck, like a tortoise disappearing into its shell. Your shoulders are also the part of your body that 'shoulder' all your personal burdens

Your Control Centre is your head and neck. Your neck is the major channel through which your brain communicates with the rest of your body, continually mediating between thoughts and feelings. Your mind operates mostly in the unconscious state. Learning to become more mindful is a process of becoming awake, conscious and in control of your mind, rather than your mind being in control of you.

So how well did you do? Did you intuitively know where your moving, being, doing and control centres were located within your body?

As Your MindBody Journey progresses, you'll get to visit each of these body centres in turn and discover the secrets that each part of your body can reveal to you. For now, here's a simple way to prepare yourself for Your MindBody Journey.

The Power Of Positive Posture

We're going to play around with posture again, but instead of pretending to be confident or unconfident you're going to start becoming aware of your natural, everyday posture.

To do this you need to be standing up, maybe in front of a mirror, but certainly somewhere where you are free to have a good look at your body. Notice your posture. It expresses very clearly who you are and what you think. What can you see?

Are your shoulders rounded bracing yourself in fear? Or are your shoulders relaxed and open and feeling confident in who you are? Are your arms open and embracing life with all its ups and downs? Or are you closed to life with your arms always folded and your shoulders habitually up towards your ears? Does your body feel flexible or inflexible and whichever it is, how is that tendency reflected in your personality?

If you lack in confidence or you feel fear regularly, then your body will withdraw and retreat. Your shoulders will droop and your head will bow and your arms will naturally fold over your vulnerable areas, such as the heart and lungs. You become like the tortoise retreating into its shell. Yet if you feel confident and don't feel fear, then the opposite will happen, your chest and arms will open and you'll hold your head up high. Your posture may show very subtle signs of your personality, perhaps barely noticeable, however they will be there if you look.

Every aspect of your posture has a hidden message that can reveal your inner truths and it takes time to get really familiar with the terrain. So to make it easy for you to start reading your own posture, we're going to focus on two distinct posture/personality types.

We will call these postures the red light reflex and green light reflex. As you read the descriptions for these posture types, see which one resonates most with you and then we'll do an exercise to help you work out if you are red or green.

Is Your Posture Red Or Green?

The **Red Light Posture** has an anterior tilt (i.e. the pelvis is tucked under) which will create a flat back and weak back muscles, tight abdominal muscles, tight hamstrings, round shoulders and leg muscles that are tight and rigid. This is a fear based posture and is usually a sign that you may be a little afraid of life.

When you have perpetual, fearful thoughts, your body starts to draw inwards for protection. There will be a 'holding back' from life. Your thoughts will be more fear based and come from the past. In extreme cases of this posture, there can be a tendency towards blocked sexual expression and a repression of, or a holding on to, your sexual feelings.

And because the energy is not flowing freely within the body, problems can include frequent leg injuries, bladder irritability, abdominal tension, lower back pain and tension headaches and gynaecological problems.

The **Green Light Posture** (lordosis) features a postural tilt, which means the pelvis tilts outwards. A person with the green light posture has an extreme curvature of the lower spine and is likely to have a tight lower back which is usually accompanied by weak and extended abdominal muscles. The quadricep muscles in the thighs will also be tight and the hamstrings are usually weak.

In this posture, the head is often thrown forward so sore muscles in the neck are a common complaint. This posture type is usually found in people who are open to life but in extreme cases can be an impatient, hyperactive doer, who is always in a hurry. This posture indicates a tendency to try and jump ahead of yourself in life and be in too much of a hurry to 'get there'. Your thoughts may be more future based and you tend not to live in the present moment. Or your mind is telling you to go forward, but you can't quite make that step, creating a forward leaning posture and tight sore leg muscles.

Exercise #3:
Testing Your Postural Reflexes

If you're not sure whether you tend towards the green or red light reflexes, here's the exercise to help you work this out.

Stand sideways in front of a full-length mirror if you have one. Firstly tilt your pelvis under, then outwards and repeat this tilt back and forth action a few times. Now go back to your normal standing position. Do your hips naturally default back to the green light posture (bottom out) or a red light posture (hips tucked under).

If you are still not sure, stand with your back against a wall with your feet two inches away from the wall. Now lean back slowly until your body touches the wall. What part of your body touched the wall first? Was it your buttocks or your shoulders? If it was your buttocks then it is an indication you are more green light, if it was your shoulders first, then it indicates you are perhaps more red light.

If your shoulder blades and buttocks touched the wall at the same time, then your posture is probably more healthy and neutral. Now practice leaning back and adjusting your posture so your buttocks and shoulder blades touch the wall at the same time. When you feel you have mastered this then move away from the wall and start walking in this corrected position. How does this feel? What does your old posture and new corrected posture say about you?

The Tale Of The Stuck Up Madam

During one of my MindBody workshops, a woman called Anna discovered she had a severe red light posture, with her hips tucked under.

We did a walking exercise to discover where the centre of gravity was in her body. Anna was walking very slowly, with her shoulders hunched and her eyes fixed on the floor. Obviously a posture of someone who isn't very confident!

I was working with her using some techniques to help her correct her posture, but she felt very uncomfortable when she tried to straighten her spine and think tall. I asked her why she didn't feel comfortable about having a more confident upright posture, she instantly replied, 'because everyone will think I'm a stuck up snob who's too big for her boots!'

She was very determined that this is how people would view her and there was no way she wanted to appear that way. 'Why do you think people would think this?' I enquired. She then went into great detail about an 'awful' girl in her class at school who was a 'nasty stuck up little madam,' who was really tall and used to walk around as if she had a pole stuck up her backside, ordering people about and saying cruel things.

Anna was bullied by this girl and ever since then she has unconsciously linked an upright posture, to being 'stuck up', cruel and bullying. Once Anna was aware of this and we worked on reprogramming her MindBody into believing that good posture represented health, grace and wisdom, she was able to walk tall again.

This is typical example of how the thoughts we think can create the body we embody and help to shape the life we live.

Does Your Body Have A Split Personality?

Another way to explore your body and discover more about yourself is to look out for 'body splits'. Some people have obvious 'identity splits' in their body where the top half is bigger or more developed than the bottom half, or vice versa.

You might know of someone who has a well-built torso, shoulders and arms but tiny stick-like legs. This body type often goes with a personality of someone who's very out going and has no problem expressing themselves verbally, with much gesturing of the arms and hands. However, they may be quite 'ungrounded' with insecure foundations in their home, family or work life. This would indicate that their life force is being expressed and is flowing healthily in their top half, but not in the lower part of their body.

Then we have the opposite split, someone with a tiny top half, with a small chest, thin arms and often rounded shoulders, but with legs and hips that are quite chunky and solid. This would indicate someone who doesn't express themselves freely, verbally or in their actions, however they are stable and grounded and are often 'home birds'.

There are also splits across the body from left to right.

The left side of the body expresses our feminine nature. These qualities are nurturing, receptive, intuitive, passive, creative, imaginative, the nature of 'being'. The right side of the body expresses our masculine qualities. These are logical, single minded, giving, active, linear, the nature of 'doing'.

The right side of the brain controls the left side of the body and the left side of the brain controls the right side of the body. You may have heard of the expression, 'he's so left brained' or 'she's so right brained' meaning that they are more 'typically male' or 'typically female' in the way they think and behave.

The masculine and feminine principles can express themselves equally within our body, regardless of whether we are male or female. If we are more dominant or dormant in either the masculine or feminine qualities, then an imbalance of this natural energy flow (known in Eastern cultures as 'yin and yang') can get disrupted. We see evidence of it in our health, showing up as issues in our bones, muscles, organs on the one side of the body only.

When the right and left sides of your brain are working in harmony, you find it easy to take a creative idea or an intuition from your right brain and use your left brain to support this idea and turn it into action, bringing the imagination into form in the process.

But if your intuition and your heart want to do one thing, and your brain butts in giving you all the excuses as to why it's a bad idea, then you will experience internal conflict. Some people say that the modern disease is that we are too governed by the active, masculine, left-brained, "doing" side of our character and don't value the receptive, feminine, right-brained tendency to just "be".

What do you think you need more or less of in your life? More doing, more being or a better balance of both?

Now you are becoming more aware of your posture, your MindBody language and the way your body has embodied all the thoughts that you think about yourself, you may notice yourself observing other people's postures. This is a good sign that you are coming more fluent in the language of the Mind-Body. Next time you're in a public place, see if you can spot the difference between people who are feeling fearful and unconfident, to the people who are feeling trusting and confident. Just try not to stare too much!

Your Energetic MindBody

As you're now becoming familiar with the map of your body, with its centres and splits, it's time to add another layer of detail. Not only do you have a physical anatomy, but you also have an energetic anatomy. Both are interrelated and the health of your energetic anatomy, affects the health and wellbeing of your physical anatomy.

You have a wide and complex set of energy systems running through your body, like contour lines on a map, which include meridians, chakras and your aura. This energy system is constantly evolving and changing in each and every moment, depending on how you are thinking and feeling. It is an integral part of your MindBody system.

We are trained to look at the physical body when something goes wrong with our health, but most of the time the issues originate from your energy body. Any imbalance within your energy system, caused by your thoughts, emotions and behaviour, can't help but show up in your physical body.

We are surrounded by a mix of electromagnetic energies of different frequencies that we can't see, some which we have harnessed like radio waves, microwaves, telephone waves, electricity waves and x-rays.

There are also the natural waves we are connected to all the time, such as the magnetic poles, light and sound waves and the electric frequencies of animals and plants. Our thoughts are also a type of energy, creating a range of different brain waves (gamma, beta, alpha, theta and delta) all of which can be observed on a machine called an EEG (which is short for an 'electroencephalograph').

Chakras, Meridians And Auras

In some Eastern traditions this 'life force' energy in and around us is called 'chi' or 'prana'. We swim in this soup of electro-magnetic energies and it interacts with our own, personal energy system.

Eastern philosophies have also identified seven 'chakras' within the body, which are spinning wheels of electric energy of different frequencies which connect your aura and your meridian system within your body. These chakras affect the flow of energy into your body. They absorb primary energy from the atmosphere (called 'chi' or 'prana') and send it along your meridian energy channels.

Every organ and body part is fed by at least one meridian energy channel that runs through the body. If the flow of the meridian is blocked it will affect the associated body part, which will inevitably result in illness. I see meridians as energy railway lines operating like our circulatory system all around the body, and the chakras are like stations where the energy rail lines pass through, regulating the energy flow. Chakras are energy transformers. Every thought and emotion we have affects our meridians and chakras.

Then there is your aura, which is an energy forcefield that surrounds, protects (a bit like your own personal ozone layer), penetrates and extends out beyond your physical body. It is an electromagnetic field, making it both electric and magnetic.

Your aura holds layers of physical, emotional, mental and spiritual elements within it. Your aura acts as a bridge or connection between the physical world and the metaphysical world and universal intelligence.

Your aura is made up of many shades of colour, which are constantly changing depending on the emotions you are experiencing. Happy and loving thoughts expand your aura while sad or angry thoughts contract your aura. Aura sizes adjust depending on the density of the population where you live. If you live in a city you will have a tighter and smaller aura. If you live in a natural rural location then your aura will be expansive. Have you ever had a radio on and notice that the sound gets distorted and crackles when you stand near it? This is your aura interfering with the radio waves.

Your aura protects you from energies outside of your body and filters the energy within your body. Your thoughts, feelings and experiences feed or deplete your energy system. This explains why your thoughts create your experiences, your electromagnetic energy system, which is a magnetic force, will literally draw to you whatever you have programmed it to attract.

Have you ever felt totally drained after visiting a friend who was depressed? They were literally draining your energy from your energy field. Have you ever had one of those days where one thing goes wrong, then everything else goes wrong?

It's not something 'out there' trying to get at you, YOU are the one who is attracting it to you. YOU are vibrating at a certain frequency of annoyance and your energy field is magnetising incidents and experiences that are annoying!

This is why the thoughts we think not only give us the body we embody, but also shape the lives we live.

KEY LESSONS FROM CHAPTER THREE

- **Become aware of your posture**

- **Changing your posture helps to change your thoughts, feelings and life experiences**

- **Learning about body centres and body splits will give you a better understanding of your own MindBody**

- **Remember, your energy body and your physical body are both part of your MindBody system**

- **Keep developing your knowledge of the MindBody language by observing other people's postures, discreetly!**

CHAPTER FOUR

Where Do You Hide Unresolved Emotions?

By now you've probably got a good understanding of how your MindBody connection works. It makes sense to most people, for example, that if you think happy thoughts and feel genuinely happy, then this happiness will be reflected in your body language and your posture.

And most people understand that if you are feeling down and stuck in a cycle of negative self talk, then one way to lift your mood is to change your body posture and send a signal to your mind that it's time to "pull your socks up", "lift your chin up" and start thinking positive thoughts again.

All of this makes perfectly good sense to most people, because we've all got embodied experience of our thoughts, emotions and body language being connected in some way. But Your MindBody Journey is much, much more than the quick fix of sticking out your chest and thinking positive thoughts until you feel better about yourself.

The secret of Your MindBody Journey goes much deeper than this. Your MindBody Journey is designed to help you discover the root cause and uncover the unconscious blocks that are holding you back from living a fulfilling, healthy life.

And the reason we struggle to overcome these mental blocks is that they're hidden from view, deep in our unconscious mind. And they are not only hidden in your unconscious mind, but they are also hidden throughout your body.

The way Your MindBody Journey works for you is to take you through a step-by-step process that helps you uncover the blocks, hidden in your MindBody, one by one, and replace them with new programming designed to help you live a life you'll love. This journey is not a temporary solution but a long term transformation.

Over the years, to protect ourselves from our vulnerabilities, we've been unconsciously covering our bodies with armouring in the form of fat or muscle, particularly in the areas where we feel most vulnerable.

Muscle and fat also store our deepest pains and fear in their soft protective tissue. The area of our body where we store most tissue, gives us an indication of where we need the most protection. Our stomachs to protect our feelings; our legs to protect us from the rug being pulled from under us; the heart and breasts from our deep pain and emotions and our arms from giving too much of ourselves.

The Tale Of The Overeating Schoolgirl

When I was a young girl in my early teens I started to get a lot of attention from the boys at school. I hated the way the boys stared at me especially as my breasts were growing so quickly and seemed to be getting bigger and bigger with every day. I started to wear baggy clothes so that I would get less attention. I didn't realise at the time, but I made an unconscious decision that if I became less attractive, I wouldn't get stared at. So I began to over eat. I ate and ate to try and cover up my body with fat to protect me from the staring eyes of the boys. This was a silly idea really because it made my breasts even bigger, but my unconscious mind was running the show. The process of over eating carried on into adulthood but, of course, I became unhappy with my weight and tried diet after diet with no success. It wasn't until I became aware of the past programming that I'd set up that I could heal the pain of my past and return to my natural weight which I've maintained ever since.

According to Dr. John Sarno M.D, a retired professor of Clinical Rehabilitation Medicine at New York University School of Medicine, everyday aches and pains in the body are not created by an old injury or old age like we often believe, the injury is a trigger, rather than a cause of the pain.

He calls this TMS (Tension Myositis Syndrome). Pain symptoms are caused by mild oxygen deprivation via the autonomic nervous system, as a result of repressed emotions and psycho-social stress. After years of treating patients with severe back pain and other major pains in the body, he discovered that the pain had in fact been created in the mind by past stresses and traumas.

The unconscious mind believed it was better to express the pain as a physical issue (usually at the site of an old injury), than to experience the emotional pain. Why? Surely feeling an emotion is better than feeling the physical pain? This is logical to us, but your emotional system is very organised and it determines how it will react and often it's not rational!

The sources of these stresses or traumas are generated from either childhood sufferings, an unrealistic drive for perfection-ism or from present life stresses. The mind has a very clever way of creating a physical distraction to trauma or stress. The mind is aware of everything that goes on in the body which includes slipped discs, whiplash, herniated discs, RSI, tennis elbow, shin splints, tendonitis, tears in the knee joint, pulled hamstrings etc. The typical triggers are accidents or incidents such as a skip or fall, sports injury, repetitive motions in your work, car accidents and so on.

As a professional sports massage therapist I have treated hundreds of injuries and I know from experience that an injury isn't always the source of emotional diversions, it can be an average muscle ache. A healthy muscle that has soreness from an activity or strain should pass in a day or two, but if the pain persists and intensifies, or the injury keeps occurring in the same place, then it is an indication that locked memory is the cause. Once this is understood you can tell the subconscious to operate differently.

What Is Your Body Holding On To?

In his book, 'The MindBody prescription', John Sarno suggests that cancer patients all have something in common within their personal characteristics. Malignant melanoma was found in patients who had a strong need to be nice and never expressed anger, worrying more about their loved ones than their selves. Ovarian cancer patients had past traumatic life events, loss or separation before the onset of cancer. Breast cancer sufferers had experienced severe heartache and grief from losing a loved one or had not been able to express maternal love, for some reason or other. Colon disorders were often linked with the repression of anger. Unexpressed grief, a feeling of hopelessness, sadness and depression are also common traits in cancer patients.

Yet the most common theme running throughout the unconscious in all Dr Sarno's TMS patients was always suppressed emotional rage. Rage is repressed in the unconscious and because we do not feel it, we cannot address or deal with it. Finding the source of the rage and not the rage itself will release the pattern.

The body speaks to us about our unresolved issues, if only we knew how to listen. John Sarno tells his patients that they must consciously think about the repressed rage and the reasons for that rage (even if they don't believe they are holding on to any rage). This effort of thinking is a counter attack, an attempt to undo the brain's strategy. He suggests you talk to your brain, tell your brain you know what it's up to and that the physical pain is harmless and that you know that all it's trying to do, is to protect you from repressed rage.

The idea is that you thank your brain for protecting you, but also being clear that this strategy can no longer go on. John says you should ask the brain to increase the blood flow to the tissues of the area of the pain to kick start the healing. He suggests listing all the pressures in your life at the moment which all contribute to your inner rage.

When you have understood and eliminated the root cause of the pain and changed the unconscious mind's reaction to your emotional state, the pain will cease. In other words, once you feel your emotional pain, the physical pain will go.

The Tale Of The Perfect Man

One of my clients was a bodybuilder called Justin who came to me because of a torn shoulder joint ligament. I noticed he was quite obsessed with how he looked and after a few private sessions with Justin, he discovered that he was unconsciously trying to obtain perfection. He wanted to have the 'perfect body' so that everyone would relate to him as the 'perfect man'.

He had a disturbing childhood with an abusive father, which made him dislike men and the masculine energy in general. After further discovery he revealed that he hated men and what they represented, and because he was a man, he hated himself. Therefore if he became the image of a 'perfect man' others would love him. What he was really trying to do was love and accept himself and the only way he felt he could do this was physically mould and shape himself into the image of a 'perfect man'.

This of course didn't work and he was destroying his body the more he worked out to become the 'perfect man'. We had quite a few sessions pealing off the layers of hurt and pain that he had locked under his armour. When Justin finally realised that he was loved regardless of how he behaved or looked, the gym obsessions became less and his self-consciousness decreased. He started to feel sorry for his body and all the suffering he had caused it. He also had to forgive his father for all the abuse, knowing that he too was abused as a child.

Exercise #4:
How Your Thoughts Shape Your Posture

Your posture not only shapes and moulds your muscles, but also your mood, your attitude and your personality. Here is a quick but effective MindBody exercise which demonstrates how your thoughts and emotions effect your body.

Stand comfortably. Tune in to your whole body. How does it feel right now? Sluggish? Energised? Tired? How does this relate to your life right now? Now Imagine you are in an extremely desirable situation where you are really happy being. It might be an image of a favourite place of yours, or you are with a person you love. Tune into your body. How does it feel? How do you feel? Is there any tension in your body? Check your heart rate and your breathing. Breathe and let that image go.

Now imagine yourself in a very undesirable situation, you are somewhere you really don't want to be. It might be a past, unpleasant experience or it might be of a fear you might have. How does your body feel now. Tune into your legs, thighs, ankles. Is there any tension? Check your heart rate and your breathing. How different does your body feel from the first image? If you have constant fearful thoughts, you can imagine what effect these negative thoughts have on your body over a period of time.

Every thought we have affects all of our body centres and the organs within that area. If you have a health problem or issue in your body then it is an indication that you are not expressing the personality of the corresponding body centre into action. Because there is no energy flow or expression in this area, it will create stagnation and stagnation will create blocked energy. You can unblock the plug and bring an energy flow back to any part of the body at any time. The key is to discover what mindset you hold that created the block in the first place. This is all part of Your MindBody Journey.

So, whatever is going on for you with your health or with your life, your answers are always there, depending on whether you want to hear them. The clues are in the language and words that you regularly use.

KEY LESSONS FROM CHAPTER FOUR

● Every thought we have affects all of our body centres and the organs within that area

● If we stop listening to our thoughts long enough to listen to our body, we'll begin to discover the impact our thoughts are having on our body

CHAPTER FIVE

Your MindBody Language

In this chapter, you'll make your final preparations for Your MindBody Journey. By now you'll have a good understanding of the territory we're about explore and you just need a little help with the language barrier before you begin.

You may not know it, but you are already fluent in MindBody language. You've been speaking it all your life, as every thought you've thought and every word you've spoken has been heard by your body---you just didn't realise that your body was listening and responding.

Your body takes your words and thoughts quite literally and manifests what you speak of. Because of the way your Mind-Body works, your body is essentially a solidified version of your mind. Any physical ailments you have are a physical expression of your mental suppression.

We've already looked at the way general thoughts and feelings like 'I'm stuck' and 'I'm scared' are reflected in our general posture. Well sometimes we also address our thoughts and words to specific parts of the body without even realising it.

Are any of these sayings familiar to you?

Feet words: 'You get right under my feet'; 'I've got cold feet'; 'I've fallen head over heals'.

Leg words: 'I want to stand my ground'; 'I can't stand it'; 'I need to put my foot down'; 'I'm down on my knees';

Buttock words: 'He's a tight arse'; She's full of shit'; 'You're anally retentive'; 'You're a pain in the arse'.

Back words: 'I'm constantly bending over backwards'; 'I'm holding back'; 'Don't turn your back on me'; 'You put my back up'; 'Get off my back';'I'm going backwards'; 'You're spineless'.

Neck and shoulder words: 'You're a pain in the neck'; 'I'm shouldering the burden'.

Arm and hand words: 'Keep something at arms' length'; 'elbow your way through'; 'I can't handle it'.

Face words: 'Saving face'; 'I can't face it'.

Organ words: 'You get right on my nerves'; 'That was nerve wracking'; 'I'm a nervous wreck', 'You are heartless'; 'You broke my heart'; 'I'm losing heart'; 'My heart isn't in it'; I refuse to see' (eyes); 'I refuse to hear' (ears); 'I need to get this off my chest'; 'You took my breath away' (lungs); 'You have a sharp tongue'; 'I'm biting my tongue'; 'You get right under my skin'.

Because your body believes every word you say, what you put in is what you get back, just like programming a computer. Most of the time we are not mindful of the thoughts and words we habitually use to tell ourselves and others how we feel, but our body is listening to every word which is why the thoughts we think eventually manifest in the body.

Your body (and your life) is shaped by the language you consciously and unconsciously use and you can literally 'sentence' yourself to a life of poor health if you don't undo any negative programming you've set up in your MindBody.

Mind Your Body Language

One of my clients was a businessman who worked himself "to the bone" and every time he came home at night he would say to his family, 'I'm shattered'. One day he didn't arrive home from work. He was involved in a head on collision with another car and almost every bone in his body was shattered. This was a serious wake up call for him and after his long slow recovery, he knew he would never go back to working too hard with long hours like he did before.

Sometimes accidents and traumas in our lives are blessings in disguise, as they push us back on track. But we don't have to wait until our body is broken and have to literally pick up the pieces. Whenever you have any kind of injury, illness or dis-ease it's a great opportunity to ask yourself what this condition is trying to tell you. What have you been saying to yourself, consciously or unconsciously, to create this reaction in your MindBody.

Here are some examples of the perpetual unconscious thoughts/phrases that can create specific medical conditions:

Diabetes: 'There's no sweetness in my life'.

Dermatitis/Acne: 'Stop picking on me'. 'I'm itching to get away'; 'You get right under my skin'; 'It's eating away at me', 'You make my skin crawl'.

Hay fever: 'You're irritating me'; 'My life is irritating me'.

Scoliosis (curvature of the spine): 'I don't express what I really think and I'm never straight with people'.

Dandruff: 'They think I'm flakey'.

Indigestion: 'This is hard to digest'; 'I can't stomach it'; 'it's eating away at me'; 'I haven't got the guts'.

Dental problems: 'Grin and bare it'; 'Sets my teeth on edge'; 'Grit my teeth'; 'Stiff upper lip';'Tight lipped';'Chew things over'.

Sore throat: 'This is hard to swallow'; 'The words get stuck in my throat'; 'The truth hurts'.

Alopecia: 'I'm tearing my hair out'.

Vomiting: 'I'm sick and tired of it'.

Headaches and migraines: 'It's giving me a headache'; 'I need that like a hole in the head'; 'It blew my mind'.

Constipation: 'I'm holding on'; 'I can't let go'. **Diarrhoea:** 'I want to run away'.

Broken limbs: 'I need a break'; 'I'm at breaking point'; 'Give me a break'.

Cystitis or kidney problems: 'You piss me off'.

The Tale Of The Pissed Off Girlfriend

Over the years I've learnt from personal experience that the problems that manifest in my body are, more often than not, shaped by the thoughts I've been thinking and the life I've been living.

There was a stage in my life when I had a bout of kidney infections while I was in a relationship with a man who constantly 'pissed me off!'. Every time I held onto these 'pissed off' thoughts a kidney or urinary tract infection would always follow. It wasn't until I resolved the issues I had with him and stopped being so 'pissed off' that the infections stopped.

I believe that if we don't listen to the whispers and don't listen to our inner guidance, then we will have to listen to the shouts! Which is another reason why it is so important to listen to our body language!

Once I realised this and the penny finally dropped, I went on my own MindBody Journey. I needed to resolve my issues around my work and to finally listen to my calling and my true direction in life. I also needed to heal the unresolved childhood hurts and upsets that constantly showed up in the form of relationships with men who kept 'pissing me off'.

Once I was finally clear on my direction in life and once I took responsibility for my relationship issues and was clear on what I truly wanted in a partnership, it was only then that my health improved, the kidney infections stopped and I finally found my soul mate.

Now that you are familiar with the body centres, posture types, your electromagnetic anatomy and the power of your Mind-Body language, here is an exercise to help your body communicate to with you. Read this exercise first, then take yourself through the process, or have someone read it to you.

Exercise #5:
How To Listen To Your Body Talk

Lay down or get into in a relaxed sitting position. Close your eyes and take a few long deep breaths to relax the body. Notice how you start to feel heavier and heavier and more relaxed with each out breath.

Bring your awareness to your body. You can feel the weight of your body as it touches the chair or floor. You are aware of your legs and how relaxed they feel. You notice your heart beating in your chest. You are aware of your tummy rising and falling with every breath. You focus all your attention internally.

After a few minutes, notice what part of the body is calling to you. A part of your body wants your attention. Where has your inner eye been naturally drawn to? Is it in your moving centre (hips legs and feet)? Your being centre (torso and back)? Your doing centre (your shoulders arms and hands)? Your control centre (your head, neck and mind)?

Once you are drawn to a particular part of your body, bring all your attention to this area. If you feel discomfort in this area, notice any thoughts or feelings you have about this part of your body. Describe it to yourself. Ask your body, 'What is this discomfort trying to teach me?' If this part of the body had a voice, what would it say to you right now? Tune into any words or phrases that might come up.

Be still and listen. Do the words relate to your life right now or do they relate to past issues and concerns that you haven't yet let go of? Be aware of any thoughts or memories that might crop up. What does your body need to help you feel better?

Now imagine how your body would feel if it had no worries, no anxieties, no pain, no stress, no complaints, no health problems, no pain or discomfort and no fears. Allow your entire system to feel how that would feel. Focus all your attention on how it would feel if you were completely free from pain and discomfort. How different does your body feel now? Let this feeling increase. Feel it in your entire being. Allow it to spread wider and deeper. Bring that feeling into your reality, because this is the real you without your created fears, worries and troubled mind.

This is your true self. It has always been there and it is always there, all you have to do is tune in to it. Breathe, let go of any negative thoughts and feelings you are holding onto and open your eyes. Now notice how you feel.

Did you uncover any insights regarding your health or your life? Does your body now feel more relaxed and free? Was there any resistance to this exercise? Did your brain want to tell you another story of how your body should feel? Did your mind sabotage this process? If so, is this a familiar pattern with you? Why do you think this is? Write down any answers.

Your MindBody Connection And Illness

Illness and disease are your body's way of telling you that something isn't working. Rather than seeing your illness or disease as an enemy, see it as an opportunity to wake up to whatever isn't working in your life. The hidden gift of your ailment is guiding you back to your true self. So coming to terms with it is your first step, because whatever you fight against will fight back.

The more serious the illness, the greater the inner issue is and often it is caused by a trauma from your past that hasn't been discharged. Your body is very smart and it will do anything to try and protect you from the emotional pain you don't want to deal with. So you may unconsciously create an illness or disease as an avoidance strategy to prevent you from having to confront a longstanding issue that you don't want to take responsibility for. Do you honestly believe you deserve to be well and healthy? If not why not? What part of you believes you deserve to be ill?

When you have learnt to yield to your illness, as opposed to resisting it, then you can see it in a new perspective. You will be able to see how the thinking and feeling patterns you have created are manifesting in your body. The great news is that as you were the one who created this programming, you can also deprogram these patterns and create new, healthier more resourceful thoughts and feelings, that help you create the life you want to live.

There is more and more evidence of people being diagnosed with serious diseases or terminal illnesses, only for them to spring back to full health a few months later. Many scientists and doctors in the past have been baffled by these impossible recoveries which seem to defy the rules of science.

How can we explain such miracles? Easy, it's all in the mind. Because your body believes every word you say, when you tell your body it's sick (or a doctor does) then you will get sick, you become your own living prophecy. The same can be true in reverse. If you believe you are fit and well, then your body believes it and then you become fit and well.

There has been much evidence of the placebo effect, for example, where two patients have the same illness. One person has been given a pill to cure them and the other has been given a pretend pill made from sugar and water. Both patients have been told they have been given a drug that will cure them. They both get better.

This is because their mind believes they will get better   because they have been told they will. It isn't just wishful thinking, scientists have now proven that when we believe we are taking a drug, but in fact it's a placebo, the brain lights up as if it was really taking the drug and produces its own natural chemicals. Some experts say that one third of medical healings are now due to the placebo effect.

Your Mind Can Heal Your Body

In David Hamilton's book called, 'How your mind can heal your body', he talks of an experiment that was done with patients with Parkinson's disease. They were given a placebo drug but were told they were given a remedy for Parkinson's. As a result, all the patients were able to move better.

Brain scans of the patients proved that the area of the brain that controls movement was activated and dopamine was actually produced. The same research was carried out giving placebos for lots of different conditions and illnesses and the results were the same.

The brain would produce a natural drug that was tailor made to combat that particular illness and the patient became well. When you believe something, chemicals are produced in the brain to heal exactly what you believe should happen. Chemicals are produced because of your beliefs. This is mind over matter in its truest sense.

The same placebo rule applies if you believe you are sick, but in fact you aren't, then you are more than likely to become sick. Chemicals will be released by your brain to attack the imaginary disease, creating autoimmune response mechanisms which will attack a perfectly healthy body. So people who continually speak of disease invariably attract it.

Continual criticism produces rheumatism, as continual unharmonious thoughts cause unnatural deposits in the blood which settle in the joints. False growths are caused by jealousy, hatred, fear and an unforgiving nature. Every dis-ease is caused by the mind not being at ease. For some people this can be life-saving information because once you realise you are creating the illness, you can also cure it!

Illness In Babies And Children

Some people ask me that if our health and lives are manifestations of our thoughts and feelings and locked up emotions, then what about babies who were born with defects; children with tragic illnesses or even pets with terminal disease.

This is not an easy question to answer because most people naturally want to blame something or someone for such illness and disease. However if you can look at a bigger picture and a wider view, then the answers are never black or white.

I believe because we are sensitive energy beings, then we can pick up energy that doesn't belong to us. Children are very open and absorb everything around them to learn and grow. This means they are extra vulnerable to the energies around them, particularly from their parents.

If a mum or dad sends out over protective fearful thoughts or feelings, or projects their own health worries or fears on to the child, then these fears are picked up and absorbed by the child. This then becomes their unconscious programming of fears, phobias and health issues, and so illness or accidents will be attracted to them through their energy field.

This also applies to babies in the womb, negative energy can be absorbed into them from their mothers and the levels of cortisol (stress hormone) in their system is then setup before they are even born.

Other theories suggest that sick children are expressing or healing dynamics from an ancestral past. If you are willing to look at an even bigger picture, then some illnesses, fears and programming are bought forward from their time before birth, the programming is bought forward from their soul or from a past life that their soul previously experienced.

These ideas may or may not resonate with you, and your intuition is the best guide to help you find your own truth when exploring such questions.

Understanding Your Illnesses

The best way for you to understand why a particular illness or disease has manifested in your body is to look at the area of the body where the disease is and then to look at its function.

For example, the function of the liver is to filter waste to prevent your body from becoming toxic. If you have jaundice or a problem liver, it could perhaps relate to your perpetual toxic thoughts.

The function of your heart is to pump oxygen to your body keeping all your organs and cells active, healthy and alive. If you close down your heart, you restrict the natural flow of your life force to all your vital organs. You become stingy, restrictive and hard-hearted, resulting in an aneurysm or a heart attack.

The joints in your body make movement easy and flexible. If you have problems in your joints, have you become inflexible and un-spontaneous in nature?

If you suffer from congestion, then you may be a hoarder of things. Congestion of things in your life can reflect congestion in your body.

Our skin is the biggest organ in the body and acts as a protective layer, so if you have skin disorders it can relate to feelings of your protection being taken away and can be triggered by loss or separation from a loved one. If you suffer from itchy or inflamed skin, then ask yourself who or what is getting under your skin? Who or what is causing you irritation?

Allergies are also set up in the MindBody to keep you safe from perceived danger. This sometimes can be linked back to a past trauma that triggered the problem. For example, if you were told off while eating a peanut, it can set up an allergic reaction in the future.

The Tale Of The Redundant Woman

A lady came to me who had been diagnosed with cancer of the appendix. Throughout a MindBody consultation with her I noticed that she repeatedly used the same key word to describe things. The word she used was 'redundant'. All her children had left home and she felt 'redundant' as a mother, she was made 'redundant' from her job, she was worried about her son who had also just been made 'redundant', she felt 'redundant' as a wife as her husband worked away a lot.

She said to me, 'Why have I got cancer of the appendix when I am so conscious of my health? I exercise and I eat healthily, why is this happening to me?' I was sad that she felt so helpless, so I asked her what she thought the function of the appendix was. She replied, 'Well there is no function of the appendix, it has been proved that the appendix is redundant.'

She looked at me and I saw the realisation cross her face as she made the connection between her symptom and her mindset. Her resolve was to start filling up her life with doing useful things, to help bring back a sense of purpose, satisfaction and fulfilment into her life. She started volunteer work at her local cancer charity shop and she became a part time teaching assistant at her local school.

A year later she came to see me and told me she no longer felt redundant and she also no longer had cancer.

Exercise #6:
Uncovering The Cause Of Your Illnesses

Your body will tell you everything you need to know, so if you have any kind of ongoing or recurring illness, disease or complaint and you want to find the root cause of it, then this next exercise is for you.

Check that you wont be disturbed. Set an intention that your unconscious will communicate with your conscious mind.

Breathe deeply and close your eyes and focus on the part of your body that is causing you the problem. See this part of your body as a friend that you want to help. Talk kindly and gently to your body as you ask it some questions.

Allow your ill health to talk to you as if it is sharing all its troubles with you. Ask why has it come into your life? What is it you need to know? What advantages does it gain by being there? What might be the downside for it to be healthy again? Ask what you can do to meet its needs in a more healthy way? Now ask what changes you need to make, within yourself and in your life, for it to become healthy and happy.

Once you have all the answers you need, thank your illness for being honest and helpful and send it your love. Make sure you reassure the part of you that is your illness by saying, 'all is well, you are safe.' Now make a promise to your illness and your self to make the changes suggested.

KEY LESSONS FROM CHAPTER FIVE

● Your thoughts and words have the power to sentence you to life of good health or poor health

● When you learn to listen to the messages your Mind-Body is sending you, it can help reveal the unconscious messages you have been sending to your body

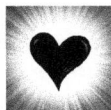

PART TWO: Your Body

OK, by now you will have a really clear picture of the way your mind, your body and your life are seamlessly interconnected. You will have a better understanding of how your thoughts, conscious and unconscious are responsible for your health and life experiences. You are probably eager to discover what hidden secrets your body is desperate to reveal to you.

So, are you ready to go on Your MindBody Journey?

It is now time to go deeper, to listen and to understand your unconscious messages and to release yourself from repeated, unhelpful patterns that no longer serve you. You will be clearing away inner obstacles that block your natural rhythms, so that your MindBody can do what it does naturally---heal itself.

You have nothing to fear, you are simply going to liberate yourself from the old patterns that don't represent the real you. It is perhaps important to remind yourself that you are not trying to get somewhere or to change things that are external to you, but rather you will be removing the walls and barriers to allow your true healthy self to shine through.

Many people experience the MindBody Journey as a process of shedding layer after layer of old conditioning. You will be stepping out of your old skin and becoming the person you know you're meant to be.

Set your intention

When you do the exercises and meditations, it will be a special time for you. Value this special time and honour yourself by taking a few steps to prepare yourself. I would suggest that each time you read a new section or do any of the exercises, turn off your phone and make it clear to anyone who shares your space that you are not to be disturbed for the next 20 minutes or so.

When I run my courses and before people arrive, I light a candle, clear the space with beautiful smells, I set an intention for the group and ask my unseen friends into the space to help guide me and the group to get their individual answers. You can do the same yourself, or do whatever works for you to prepare.

You will need a pen or pencil to write down your answers when you are prompted. Only by writing words down will you get clarity regarding your unconscious. It is important to keep your answers as you will be asked to refer to them at the end of the book, so if you'd prefer not to write in this book, you may want to write the questions on a separate piece of paper as you go, or photocopy the questions when you get to them and write your answers next to them.

You will find some of the exercises more relevant to you than others. Be your own guide to know what area of your body and what exercises and meditations need more time and attention.

Throughout your journey, you may get images pop into your head of past events that you had completely forgotten about! This is an indication that they were key moments in your life that were a catalyst to your programming. You are bringing the unconscious to the conscious, so take note of these memories and messages as they are all relevant. Also you may find you dream more, again take notes of the things you remember. I would also strongly suggest you have a clear intention of what you want to achieve from your MindBody Journey, because when you have a clear intention, you will get your answers.

So let's begin.

We will start at the bottom of your body and work our way up.

CHAPTER SIX

Your Moving Centre

Your Feet

We're going to start your MindBody journey with your feet. Remember, this is the first time you will prepare yourself to focus on a specific part of your body, so be mindful of the routine you are creating.

Paying attention to this process will help you to develop a personal ritual that enables you to make the most of each session as you take this journey of self discovery, one step at a time, up through your body, starting with your feet.

Whatever you do to prepare yourself for your MindBody practice, it's a good idea to take a moment to remind yourself of the personal intention you created in Chapter 5.

As you do this, be sure to let go of any other thoughts or concerns you may have just for now. It's okay to let go of these thoughts, if they are important, they'll come and find you when you are ready to attend to them again.

We'll start with some interesting information about feet in general before exploring what your feet say about you.

A Journey To The Bottom Of Your Sole

From a MindBody perspective, your feet connect you to the earth and so they represent how grounded you are in your life. Are you confident standing up for yourself or can you be a bit of a pushover?

You use your feet to provide you with stability and support, so any imbalances you have in your feet can throw everything off centre, not just in your body but also in your life. Your feet and ankles can also represent the ease and certainty of your direction in life. Are you clear where you're going or are you stuck or unsure of the next step to take?

Facts About Your Feet

Did you know there are 26 bones and 33 joints in each foot? On an average day, most people will take around 10,000 steps. Our feet work hard all day, every day, carrying the full weight of our body, wherever we want to take it. No wonder most people love a great foot massage.

If you're familiar with the ancient art of reflexology, you'll already know that your feet are a map of your body. According to reflexologists, every part of your body, inside and out, has a corresponding point on the soles of your feet.

The theory is, that if you have any sore points on your feet, then it indicates an excess or lack of chi energy in the corresponding part of the body.

Taking A Stand For What You Want

When I was in my twenties, I always used to get problems with aching legs. I just couldn't rest them as they felt so uncomfortable, especially at night. It turned out I had something called restless leg syndrome.

As the name suggests, it was a very restless stage in my life as I was unsure and unclear about what direction I should be taking. Looking back, I now realise that my restless mindset, was manifesting, not just in my body, but in my life.

Every job or relationship I had just didn't feel right for me. I couldn't 'stand it' and I wanted to 'run away'. But I carried on regardless because I was too concerned about money and security to listen to my heart and make a change.

So the energy of wanting to run away was never expressed and it remained within me, creating the restless leg syndrome. I needed to stop and listen to the message my body was sending me and take action to either accept my current circumstances or be responsible for taking a new direction in life.

This is how your MindBody connection works, it sends you important messages from your subconscious that need your attention. Unfortunately, I didn't realise this at the time so the messages got louder and louder until I had to pay attention when I had an accident and broke my ankle.

It was then I realised that these constant, restless, 'I can't stand it' thoughts had come true. I could no longer stand—literally! Being forced to spend six weeks in plaster, on crutches, was exactly what I needed to make me slow down and take time to decide what I really wanted to do with my life.

Of course it would be a lot easier if I'd listened to my body in the first place, rather than waiting until I broke my ankle! It was a painful and embarrassing way to learn an important lesson.

So now it's your turn to start listening to the messages that your body is trying to tell you as you take the first step on your MindBody journey.

Every Journey Starts With One Small Step

As you get to know your body better throughout the course of this book, you'll probably notice that you are becoming more aware of the way you operate. This is how the MindBody connection will work for you. By taking time to consider different parts of your body one at a time, you will begin to uncover the thoughts, feelings and unconscious beliefs that shape your life.

So let's find out what your feet reveal about you, your life and your personality. Remember, don't think too much about what's true or not, listen to your body and feel what's true for you. Leave the parts that aren't helpful to you right now behind, and follow what feels true for you in this moment and just see where it takes you. Be sure to make a note of any insights or observations you have. Take off your shoes and socks (that's of course if you have them on!) and read through the descriptions of different types of feet below and notice which apply to you.

Different Types Of Feet

Flat Feet: these can indicate a lack of grounding, never quite putting roots down and never standing still. If you have flat feet you would probably prefer to skim over the surface of things, never fully committing to one thing or another. You are a 'flitter' who probably lacks a firm footing in life. Flat feet can also indicate weaknesses in the kidney and intestines.

High Arches: these are the opposite of flat feet and can be accompanied by a tendency to clutch the ground with your toes and heels. People with high arches often have clear boundaries between private and public life and because of this may be aloof and withdrawn. You are probably a private person who deals with confrontation by 'clutching' with your body and feet. Sometimes, this can be due to an unresolved issue such as an emotional crisis where you wanted to run away, but you didn't react to that emotional impulse. So now your tendency is to hold on and keep everything under control. This usually transfers up your body and can result in tight muscles in your back.

Wide Feet: You are a hard worker.

Narrow Feet: You'd rather have others run around after you.

Weight in your heels: do you lean backwards or are you heavy on your heels? The clue here is if you have holes in the heels of your socks! This means you have a tendency to dig your heels in with determination to help you stay in control of things. It's usually because you fear instability. You resist spontaneous situations. Often this tendency is accompanied by lower back pain and a rigid pelvis.

Weight in your toes: are you a tip-toer? Do you put most of your weight on your toes? If so, you're probably a floater, a dreamer, full of flighty ideas and never quite down to earth.

Toes: are your nails ripped and torn? This is often a sign of too much negative self talk. If the necks of your toes are long, it can be a sign of an expressive personality.

Big Toe: if the neck of your big toe is large then you may find it hard to express what you truly think in fear of judgement.

Second Toe: people whose second toe is their biggest toe are said to make good leaders.

Second and Third Toe: for some people, the second and third toes lift up and this can be a sign that you are still unsure of your direction in life.

Fourth Toe: if your fourth toe bends towards your big toe on the left foot, this may be a sign that you tend to cling to things (e.g. you are a hoarder). If this is happening on your right foot then you probably tend to cling to people.

Little Toe: can you wiggle your little toe independently? It usually means you are adventurous and need constant change and stimulation.

Clutching Toe: if your toes curl downwards like they are clutching the ground then you possibly have a rigid outlook on life, and you resist change.

Pigeon Toed: you like to follow the direction of others rather than your own direction.

Feet Turned Out: you're not sure of your physical/material direction (right foot) or your spiritual/emotional direction (left foot). You like to swap directions frequently.

Heavy Footers: you have a strong need to be grounded, to be stable and to know your direction.

Fast Walkers: you are impatient and in too much of a hurry to get to your destination in life.

Slow Walkers: You are a procrastinator.

Common Foot Problems

Do you suffer from particular foot problems? If so what is your body telling you?

Athlete's Foot: you may not be feeling accepted or you may be letting things get under your skin.

Bunions: you're not enjoying the process of life and you like to hand responsibility to others, or you allow yourself to be dominated by another.

Cold Feet: you're not loving the direction your life is going.

Clammy/Sweaty Feet: you're feeling bogged down with the detail and not seeing your direction clearly.

Smelly Feet: your direction is offensive to you!

What Are Your Ankles Saying?

Your ankles reflect the support you feel you can rely on (or not) from others and yourself. Sprained or twisted ankles indicate a resistance or lack of flexibility to the direction you are taking in life. If the strain is too great for you it can cause the energy in your ankle to buckle or twist. A swollen ankle signifies that you may be holding on to emotional energy and that you're resistant to letting go of something. A broken ankle can represent a deep conflict of the ground you are standing on and a resistance to changes in your life direction.

Take Time To Talk To Your Feet

Throughout your MindBody journey I'll be inviting you to 'talk to' and 'listen to' parts of your body. This may sound like an odd thing to ask you to do at first, but you can talk to your body because your mind and body are one and the same. Your mind doesn't have a mouth but you know that it always talks to you. Take a listen to your mind now. What is it saying?

Is it saying 'this is stupid' I can't talk to my feet?"; is it saying 'this is a great idea I can't wait to try it?'; or is it saying "I wonder what's on TV tonight?"

Our heads can tend to be filled with mindless chatter, not all of it helpful, so if we want to tap into the deeper wisdom of our MindBody we need to stop any unhelpful thoughts for a moment. So if your mind is talking to you in an unhelpful way right now, just tell it politely to "SHUT UP!" so you can listen mindfully to your body.

You already know that your body talks to you. Have you ever experienced your stomach telling you when you're hungry, for example? Do you know the difference between what your body says you need to eat and what your mind says you want to eat?

You probably do. And do you always listen to the wisdom of your body when it says 'nibble a carrot' or do you prefer to give in to your chatterbox mind when it says 'mmmm, carrot cake'? Maybe you do a bit of both?

This is a very simple example of your body talking to you and the type of conversations you're going to have on your Mind-Body journey go much deeper than a rumbling tummy.

Everything that ever happened to you is imprinted in your MindBody. So the stories that you hold in your body are a web of thoughts, feelings and beliefs that you have accumulated throughout your life and may even have been inherited from your ancestors or a past life.

The answer to every challenge you face in life can be found within, once you know how to access the wisdom of your MindBody. So when I invite you to talk to your feet and consider what they can tell you, what I am really asking you to do is listen to your whole MindBody, while focusing on a specific part.

Let's try it now.

Tune into your feet and start to listen to what your feet are trying to say. Notice what thoughts and feelings arise up as you take time to focus on your feet. As you listen to your feet, let your MindBody respond by allowing any unconscious messages that are stored in this part of you body, become part of your conscious awareness.

What do they say about you? Do you take care of your feet? What are your feet telling you about yourself and your life? Get an idea of the story your feet are telling you. Do you like your feet?

How you feel about your feet is how you feel about yourself!

Take a moment to let this sink in and when you are ready jot down any thoughts, insights and observations that arose during that test before you start the next exercise.

Exercise #7:
Finding Your Roots

Here's a simple exercise to help you find what your feet are communicating. If you want to get the most out of this exercise be sure to make time to do it from start to finish.

Start by standing with your feet slightly apart. Now keeping your feet flat on the floor see how far you can lean to the left without losing your balance. Don't bend at the waist, keep your legs straight and your torso upright. Now return to centre and do the same on the other side. Notice how your feet respond as you lean gently to one side and then lean to the other.

Now do the same leaning forwards and backwards. Again, don't bend at the waist, keep your legs straight and your trunk upright as you gently lean forwards and backwards noticing how your feet react to these movements. Now stop and look at you feet.

What have you noticed? Do your feet point in or out? Do you grip your toes to keep yourself stable? Do you dig your heals in? Do you resist it or go with the flow? When you lean from side to side and front and back, how far do you feel comfortable going? How does this relate to your personality and how stable you feel in areas of life?

Take a moment to consider what your feet are telling you about your mindset, your personality and your life.

Now, keeping your feet flat on the floor, rotate your body making a circle joining the four points that you've already leant out to---front, back, right and left. Make the circle several times noticing what happens with your feet. Then stop and rotate in the opposite direction, make a circle with your body as you pay attention to your feet. Tune into any thoughts or feelings. Are you stable and confident and in control, or do you notice that you're all over the place? Do you fear falling over? Do you avoid tripping up by remaining in your comfort zone? Do you feel a sense of support from your feet, or do you feel a bit wobbly?

Now come to stillness, close your eyes and bring all your awareness of your feet.

Can you get a sense of how your feet and ankles are FEELING in the stillness of standing? Are there any words that describe these feelings? Let your feet speak to you. Listen to the language of your feet. How do these feelings or words relate to your stability in life? Your standing in life? Your willingness to change and try a new direction?

When you're ready, stop and write down any insights, or mindsets or thoughts that you have noticed are linked to your feet or ankles. Think about your sense of security, how grounded and stable you are, your ability to stand on your own two feet, how flexible in your direction you are. Use words or phrases to capture the feelings and thoughts that arose as you focused on your feet.

Creating Positive Mantras And Affirmations

Once you've completed the exercises in this section, you should have a list of words and phrases that have come to mind as you have focused on your feet.

You may be lucky and find that everything you've written down about your feet is positive and resourceful. If however you have found that some of the language associated with your feet is negative, then it's a good idea to consider how you can rewrite the story your feet are telling you.

One way to start to reprogram any limiting thoughts, feelings and beliefs you uncover on your MindBody journey, is to create a new story for that part of your body.

Inventing positive affirmations is a great way to develop new neurological pathways that, in time, will help to create new thought patterns about yourself and your life. The more you repeat these affirmations with conviction and positive emotion, the quicker you will start to see change starting to happen.

If the story that emerged when you spoke to your feet was 'I'm stuck', for example, you could invent a new affirmation to rewrite that belief.

You might be tempted to simply write a negative version of your past story, like 'I don't want to be stuck' or 'I am not stuck'. This is unlikely to work because although your intention is good, you are bringing more focus onto the thing that you don't want.

Your unconscious mind can't process negatives like the word 'not' or 'don't want to be', so telling yourself 'I am NOT stuck' or 'I DON'T WANT to be stuck', is just the same as saying "I AM stuck" and so you end up back where you started with a different version of the same old story.

And as you probably made up that story years ago when you were a child, it really is time to let it go and create a new set of beliefs that serve you and help you to live the life you want to live as an adult.

So if you want to create a better future for yourself, try asking this question, 'If I didn't have this story about my feet (e.g. 'I'm stuck'), what new story could I create for my life that would really inspire me?' If you weren't 'stuck', for example, maybe you could create a story about 'being free' or 'going on lots of adventures' or 'trying new directions'.

Creating new thought patterns takes a little practice and one way to make your affirmations stick is to include some powerful emotions in your new mantras. So don't just say 'I'm free', say 'I love to be free' or 'I really enjoy the feeling of being free every second of every day'.

Be as creative as you like when designing your affirmation, remember this is your new life story you are writing!

Once you have written an affirmation you are happy with, repeat it to yourself several times a day or as often as you can remember. You don't have to believe the statement at first, but the more you repeat the words with feeling, the more your body will believe you.

Remember your thoughts, feelings and words will ultimately be reflected in your body and in your life and the more you practice this process, the quicker you'll get results.

My affirmation to reprogram the language of my Feet is:
....
....

The Power Of Visualisation

As you make your way through the different stages of your MindBody journey, you'll be stopping to relax at the end of each chapter to allow your new beliefs to start to take root. We'll be doing this with the aid of visualisation exercises. Visualisation is simply a form of meditation where your mind is focused on a particular task.

Before you experience your first visualisation it is important to assess how skilled you already are at visualisation. Some people think that they cannot visualise but everybody can. Can you imagine what your front door looks like? Or the inside of your car? Or the face of a friend or family member? Would you recognise any of these things or people if I showed you a picture of them? Of course you would because you can instantly picture what they look like.

The way we picture things in our mind varies from person to person. Some people see full-colour pictures; some get a feeling of what something looks like and some may even use words to describe what they are visualising.

In my experience, people who say they can't visualise are blocked by their expectation that they should be able to see bright, colourful images. This isn't always the case. The way you visualise things is perfect for you.

So imagine your front door again and notice how you picture it. However you did that is the perfect way for you to visualise things. It doesn't matter if you saw your front door in colour, in black and white, or whether you got a sense of it, or smelt it or just described it to yourself with words.

However you pictured your front door, that's the way you visualise things.

So make sure you take time to use the skills you already have and enjoy these powerful visualisation exercises. The thoughts, feelings and beliefs that you are reprogramming have been held in your body for years. It can take time to create new thought patterns and these visualisations are designed to speed up that process.

♥ Meditation #1:
Footprints In The Sand

Now it is time to enjoy your first visualisation to help you feel a sense of purpose, support and grounding in life.

If you don't have time or you decide you are already secure, grounded and are self supportive, then feel free to skip this part or come back to the meditation another time when you feel you need to. Read through it first or get someone to read it to you while you meditate.

Make sure you won't be disturbed and that you have around 15 minutes of time to spare. Sit or lay in a comfortable position with your spine straight and take in some long, slow deep breaths.

Feel your body letting go of any tension and thoughts each time you breathe out. One way to relax is called the progressive relaxation technique where you start by relaxing your feet and then bring your attention up your body relaxing each part of you, bit by bit, until you reach your face. As you do this you will notice your body sinking further and further into relaxation.

Now when you are ready, picture yourself standing alone on a big sandy tropical beach, with the sun shining. You feel a warm breeze around your body. Breathe in the warm salty air. You feel contented and at peace.

Dig your feet into the sand and feel how soft and warm it feels. The sand is made from tiny particles of ancient rocks, shells and minerals, which have been around for millions of years. That warm, yellow sand is here to support and welcome you as all your issues dissolve into the ground.

Allow your feet to sink further into the warm soft sand. Allow any tension, negative thoughts or feelings regarding your stability, security and direction in life to be absorbed into the sand. Imagine these unwanted thoughts and feelings as an energy that no longer belongs to you, as you feel it being absorbed back into the earth's elements where it will be dissolved.

Feel the wisdom, the love and the power from these ancient minerals. Feel the power of the sand, the wisdom and love from this ancient sand coming up through your feet, through your legs, up into your body and into your whole being. Feel its live, tingling, loving energy. Allow that feeling to grow, welcome the feeling. Bathe in its unconditional love for you.

You are part of this energy and its wisdom and will always be so. With this knowing, you feel a sense of strength, stability and self support. You are stable and strong and can walk through life with a sense of purpose and grounding. Feel the energy of this in the whole of your being. Feel a love and peace returning to you now.

You can get in touch with this feeling any time you wish as it is part of who you really are. You have nothing to fear. You are strong, you are secure, you are stable and you trust in yourself and your path forward.

As you bring this meditation to a close, imagine yourself stepping forward into the rest of your life, taking this feeling within you.

KEY LESSONS FROM CHAPTER SIX

● **Bring loving awareness to your feet, every small step they take carries you one step closer to your dreams**

CHAPTER SEVEN

Your Legs

In this chapter we will focus on the area of your moving centre that represents your direction of travel in life. Make sure you take a moment to focus your intention on learning whatever lessons you need to learn from this chapter, it's all about you and the direction your life is heading in.

Your legs represent and express how "grounded" you are in life. They also reflect the passage of life you have experienced so far and the direction your life is heading in right now. Legs also represent your standing in the world and therefore how others see you and relate to you. They communicate how well you are able to "stand up for yourself".

So what do your legs say about you? See if any of the descriptions below relate to you. Write down any discoveries.

Weak Legs: tend to indicate that there is a lack of energy passing through them. The lack of grounding or inability to stand up for yourself and be strong on your own. If the life force in your legs is strong, you are likely to be in touch with the practical aspects of your life and able to stand up for yourself. If the life force in your legs is weak, you may have difficulties with the practical elements of life, such as your ability to earn and deciding what direction to take. You may also find you often trip up because you are unsure of your footing. If your legs are weak you may unconsciously stiffen or brace your legs, tensing the muscles and locking the knee joint, which can result in a stiff way of walking.

Strong Legs: mean you have a stable foundation, but If your legs are too strong with over developed muscles, the energy is then too rooted in the ground, so there is little room for spontaneity or a change in direction. This can mean you tend to 'hold on' to things which are familiar and safe. You may also have a tendency for repetition, for always following the same path or direction.

Fat Legs: tend to reveal similar characteristics to strong legs, but you will perhaps be unconsciously covering up any issues to do with your stability and direction. You may feel apathetic about moving forward in your life.

Tight Lean Legs: are usually a sign that you're full of energy, a 'go getter'. However, tight legs are often unyielding so if your life force isn't flowing, your direction won't be smooth. This means you may be erratic and inconsistent in nature, so there could be a tendency for your joints to become brittle over time.

Tight Legs: If the backs of your legs (hamstrings and calves) are tight or inflexible this can relate to a fear of letting go and a need to be in control.

More generally, when there is tightness, tension or pain in your legs, this usually represents a conflict with the direction you are taking, or a sense of insecurity that the rug could be pulled from beneath you at any moment. The tension is a sign of fear, a sign you are holding on to something, a fear that if you let go and go forward, you will fall or be 'let down' in some way.

You may be holding back from where you really want to go in life. If there is doubt or resistance to the direction or movement to what's happening in your life, then your legs will try to hold back that movement. They will resist change.

Knees: your knee joints represent your ability to bend, to yield and be spontaneous. It's where you express both your pride and your humility. If you have difficulty with your knees, you may have difficulty in giving in, to surrendering and accepting a situation. Are you stubborn? Also if you resist change and have a reluctance to surrender to your direction, then your knees will feel the strain. This is all due to a lack of energy flow within the joints, which are designed to bring you flexibility.

If you have pain, weakness or stiffness in the knees, there could be an imbalance in those areas. This is all connected to your thought patterns and how you digest, assimilate and absorb your life experiences. Do you resist and hold onto old thought patterns, or do you go with the flow and embrace the new? Remember, the thoughts you think give you the life you live and the body you embody!

Right Leg: The right side of your body represents the masculine, assertive, practical aspects of your character. If there are problems in your right leg or knee then this suggests that perhaps you are not being assertive enough and you need to be more active in mental, emotional and physical activities.

Left Leg: The left side of you body represents the feminine, passive, intuitive aspects of your character. If you have a problem in your left leg or knee, this means that perhaps you are not being passive enough and need to slow down.

As you consider what your legs can tell you about yourself, take time to listen to any answers or insights or observations that rise up from your unconscious mind and be sure to make a note. When you're ready, move on to the next exercise.

Exercise #8:
How To Centre And Balance Yourself

These exercises are designed to help you 'find your centre'.

Stand in a comfortable position. Bring all your attention to the way you are standing. What muscles are working to hold you up? What muscles feel tight and over worked? Where is your weight distributed? Is it on the front of your feet or your heels?

Is the weight on the inside or outside of the foot? Now get into a position where the weight is evenly distributed in your feet and unlock your knees. Stand tall by imagining there is a piece of string attached to the centre of your crown pulling your crown up to the ceiling. The key to posture control is relaxing the neck and thinking upwards with the back easing upwards and outwards and your chest opening. Check that the muscles in your legs are relaxed.

Breathe deeply in and out from your abdomen. At the end of your out breath, very slightly engage your abdominal muscles as you push the remaining air from your lungs. This is your natural standing posture and your core muscles are supporting you. Your core is your energy centre, where your power comes from.

In Japan they call this the 'hara'. When you are centred in your hara, by which I mean your centre of gravity and your physical awareness is in your abdomen, you are centred in your being energy. You are anchored within yourself, so that no matter what chaos is going on around you, you can feel centred and stable. The more you practice this posture, the more you will feel grounded and centred in life.

Now from this centred standing position, lean forward as far as you can. Keep leaning forward until you need to take a step forward to stop you falling over. What foot went forward first? Whichever foot it was, this is your dominant leg.

Do it again to check you get the same results. If it was your left leg that went forward each time, then you are more likely to be led by your feminine energy, if it was your right leg, then you are likely to be led by your masculine energy.

The Tree Pose

If you want to become more anchored, grounded and stable, there are a couple of yoga exercises you can do to help you with this. The simplest (but often the hardest, until you've mastered it) is the modified version of the tree pose.

Again stand in a comfortable position and focus on a spot in front of you. Keep your gaze on this spot as you raise your right leg. Keep your left leg locked as if it were a tree trunk with its roots firmly anchoring you into the ground. Interlace your fingers and bring them to just under your right bended knee. Stand with your back tall and stay centred in your hara and see how long you can stay balanced on one leg until you topple.

It is important that you don't judge yourself in this exercise, cursing yourself if you can't get the balance will just make it worse. Watch what your mind is doing to sabotage your balance. The more you practice, with focus and patience, the easier the exercise will become.

Now try the other leg. Were you more stable on one leg than the other? Which leg supports you more in life? Your masculine (right) or your feminine (left)? Practice this until you feel stable, grounded and strong. When you are stable and strong within yourself, you will find you have support and stability out side of yourself. This is the universal law which is known as 'as within, so without'.

Finally, keeping your legs together, gently bend from the waist until you feel the backs of your legs pulling. How far can you go? How flexible are you in moving forward in life? Tune into the 'feel' of the stretch. How does it feel? What are the words associated with that feeling. Now open your legs wide and bend down from your waist to see how flexible the inside of your legs are. Again tune into words that might come up while in the stretches. How do your words relate to your direction in life and where you are heading? Is your foundation strong or weak?

The Tale Of The Woman Who Wouldn't Give Up

Sandy was a married woman in her late thirties who attended one of my workshops. When she did the standing on one leg exercise, she couldn't get her balance. She only managed a few seconds before she toppled over.

'What's going through your mind right now?' I asked.

She said, 'I'm annoyed with myself, I hate the way I can't get balanced' .

I asked her why she felt so unstable and she immediately replied, 'I'm always all over the place, I'm never still'.

I asked her why she was never still' and the reason she gave was, 'Because there is no time to be still'.

'Why is this? I asked and she responded 'Because if I'm still it means I've given up'.

'What is it that you've given up'? I asked sensing we were getting to the root of the issue. She sighed, then tears came into her eye's and she said, "I'll give up trying to have a baby'.

It was then she realised she was running away from her infertility issue. She hadn't even wanted to talk to her husband about it, for fear he would blame her. She was in constant 'flight mode' and running away, which made her even more unstable and insecure.

Luckily after this realisation, she opened up to her husband and together they were able to go for fertility treatment. She became a lot more grounded and stable in her mind and body, which in turn, helped her to conceive and follow her chosen path of becoming a mother.

Now you have become more familiar with your legs and knees, write down what you think they say about you. How easy is it for you to stay centred, grounded and stable? Is your foundation strong or weak? How do your legs and knees relate to your direction in life?

What can you change to bring the energy in this area into healthy balance? Can you change your thought patterns or your posture or even the direction you are taking in life?

If you found that the MindBody language of your legs is fairly negative then it's a good idea to write a positive affirmation or statement to help you create new, more resourceful thought patterns. Use the words you wrote as your starting point and create a new affirmation you can repeat every day, or as often as you feel it is needed, to help you create a new MindBody neurological pathway. Act as if you believe the statement, feel what it would feel like if you were being and living the words you have created.

Remember, the thoughts and words you create in your mind, become feelings and actions in your body, that help you create the life you want to live.

My affirmation to reprogram the language of my legs and knees is:..
....

♥ Meditation #2:
Finding Your Roots

We'll finish this section with a great visualisation to help you feel grounded, secure and stable. You can use this technique when you feel yourself being swept away in the dramas of life.

Make sure you won't be disturbed and that you have 15 minutes of time to spare. Read the meditation through first (or get someone to read it out to you) then sit or lay in a comfortable position with your spine straight and take in some deep breaths. Feel your body letting go of any tension and let any thoughts you have float away and out of your conscious awareness. Feel your body sinking further and further into relaxation with each and every breath.

In your mind's eye, picture yourself in a wide-open space. Picture in front of you a green grassy hill. Now imagine yourself walking up that hill, effortlessly and slowly walking to the top. No effort at all, you seem to be almost floating to the top. You are now at the very top and all around you is the most amazing view. Get a feeling of expansiveness and openness.

Now Imagine there is a special tree standing at the very top of the hill. Imagine what your tree looks like. Get a clear picture of what the trunk, branches, leaves look like. Is it a big strong tree? Or is it a small young tree?

Now imagine you can step right inside the tree to get a sense of what it feels like. Imagine you are that tree. Feel its strength. Feel your feet which are your roots digging deep into the earth. Going down from your feet, down, down into the earth. You feel so stable and strong. You feel so grounded, stable and secure. You are strong but yielding, so that if there was a strong wind, you would bend and take its weight. You wouldn't snap under the pressure, you would yield and surrender to your conditions. Nothing bothers you because you know you are strong and stable and you trust yourself completely.

With that sense of strength, and stability you now step out of your tree and start walking back down the hill, feeling light but strong, stable and grounded. Walking with attention, intention, purpose and direction down the hill, until you're at the bottom.

Now bring your focus back to your resting body and notice how your body is feeling now. You can get in touch with this feeling any time you wish as it is your security, your strength, your stability and your complete trust in yourself.

KEY LESSONS FROM CHAPTER SEVEN

- **Pay close attention to your legs, they represent your standing and direction in life and will let you know if you're on the right track or not**

CHAPTER EIGHT

Your Hips And Pelvis

In this chapter we will explore the root of your 'moving centre', which is your pelvis. Be sure to take a moment to prepare yourself for exploring the final part of your moving centre.

Your pelvis is the foundation upon which your entire body rests. It is the hinge which mediates between the upper and lower half of your body; the impulse behind moving forward.

If you are tight or inflexible in your pelvic area, this is where you could be stuck in moving forward in life. The pelvis is the centre of where you hold your ability to stand on our own and walk your own path, without insecurity or fear stopping you.

If you're fearful that there is nothing to move forward to, or you're afraid of where you are going, your hips will reflect this. Any stiffness or problems here indicate a fear of change, an inability to let go of the past, or a feeling of being unable to stand on your own. Emotional dependence on someone else, often relating back to our mothers, is often held in this area of the body. If you've not fully broken free of the parent-child dynamic with your mother, this may be reflected in your hips and can show up in your life as a tendency to over mother others too much.

As you focus on your hips and pelvic area, consider how you normally walk. Where does your power come from? Next time you take a walk, check your body and feel where your centre of gravity sits in your body. Are your head and shoulders leading? Are your feet and ankles? Are you walking tall or are you bowed? Notice your pace, are you a plodder or a racer? Are you a leader or a follower? Are you mindful of every step, or do you tend to be in your head? Where is your head? Are your thoughts mostly about the future or the past? If you are a clear and confident walker you will more than likely have a clear and confident mind.

Remember, our thoughts create our body and together they shape our lives.

Unfortunately most of us have got into bad walking habits. The ball and socket joints within our hips are perfectly designed so we can rotate our legs in all directions. The 'catwalk' style of walk where we move our entire body to walk has now long gone. We are too concerned about looking like a weirdo or a bit 'camp'. Therefore most of us don't move our hips fully when we walk.

We are no longer using the muscles in the way they were designed, eg: running, jumping, rotating the legs and the upper body, which were all very necessary manoeuvres to catch our evening meal in our ancient past! And because we don't use our muscles in this way, they become inflexible, they get locked and blocked and eventually seize up. This is evident in the huge demand for hip replacements.

The pelvis also holds the energy of our sexual expression. In Ken Dytchwald's classic book, Bodymind, he describes an experiment he did with a group of older people who had hip issues. After a series of daily exercises to loosen up the hips, within a week, nearly all of the group members reported an enormous amount of freed up sexual energy! As they practiced each day and limbered up the pelvic muscles, sexual feelings and desires that had lain dormant for many years became activated!

Your Buttocks

Let's get to the bottom of things (literally!) In terms of the MindBody connection, your bottom is the place where you sit on things that you don't want anyone else to see. Check your bottom muscles now. Are they unconsciously tight? Are they relaxed? If they are tight consciously relax them now and notice how different you feel and the difference in your attitude. What feelings are you holding on to and sitting on? Are you 'armouring' or blocking emotional expression? How much are you holding back and trying to ignore? Do you hold on to things and have a need to control events and people?

If you have constantly tight buttocks (I call it 'anal armour'!) then you may be holding on and not expressing certain thoughts and feelings. Or you may be holding onto basic material and survival needs and money concerns, which leads to the expression 'tight arse'. Buttocks also relate to elimination and the releasing of feelings. The experience of being potty trained as a child can have a huge effect on the rest of a person's life, especially in their ability to feel relaxed and spontaneous and fearful of the unknown and unexpected.

If you have tension in the anal region (the telltale sign is dimples in your gluteus muscles) it may mean you usually suppress your emotions and may have developed a tendency towards rigid intellectual control. It also sometimes relates to our parents and their expectations of us. Do you still feel you have to live up to their expectations? Do you feel they interfere with your decision making processes?

Exercise #9:
How To Build Your Base

To check if you have 'anal armour' tune into your pelvic region. Are your bottom and pelvic floor muscles tight at the moment? As you bring your attention to this area, breathe in and then on the out breath let all the muscles relax in this area. Did you notice if they loosened a little? Return to this exercise in a few hours time. Pick a random moment in your day to tune into this area and check again. Are your pelvic floor and buttock muscles constantly contracted?

A good way to retrain these muscles and to separate the unconscious MindBody patterning in this area, is to consciously isolate each of your inner core muscles. This includes your urethra, (the muscle that stops you from urinating) Your vaginal or penile muscles and your anus. Isolate each muscle one by one by contracting each one separately. (A small note of caution here. I would advise you not to do this exercise if you are reading this book in a public place as the facial expressions that go with this exercise can be quite expressive!)

Can you tell the difference between the muscles you are isolating? Are you holding your gluteus muscles, abdominals even lower back or jaw unconsciously while you do this? Do the muscles work independently or only together as one unit? If you cannot isolate these muscles then you will more than likely have an inflexible pelvis, blocked root and sacral chakra and very tight abdominal muscles.

If this is the case, it is likely that your creativity, feelings and actions won't spontaneously flow. The process of 'letting go' and 'going with the flow' probably won't feel comfortable or natural to you.

At this point I would like to introduce the chakra system because the health of the hips and buttocks are often related to the base and sacral chakras, which are located in this area. If you are not familiar with the seven chakras, then here is a brief explanation.

Your Chakras

In Eastern cultures, the chakras are considered to be part of your energetic anatomy as distinct from your physical anatomy. When someone is ill or 'not quite right', those who practice traditional Eastern medicine will often treat the energy body before the physical body.

There are seven main chakras in your body running up the pathway of your spine, from the base of your spine to the top of your head.

The chakras regulate the flow of energy throughout your body via the electrical network that runs through the body called meridians. The chakras connect your spiritual and etheric body to your physical body.

Each chakra in the body is linked to one of the glands in our endocrine system which produces specific hormones, so when a chakra is blocked or unhealthy, then the function of our glands and the production of these hormones will be compromised which will inevitably affect the health of our body. Underactive or overactive chakras can create a variety of issues. Underactive chakras can translate into fatigue, lethargy, weight problems, a negative attitude towards life or a lack of zest for living. Overactive chakras create other types of problems including hyperactivity, panic attacks, emotional imbalances and many other types of health issues in the physical body.

This is why it is vital our energy anatomy is clear, flowing and healthy. We will be clearing each chakra during the exercises throughout your MindBody Journey.

The Seven Chakras And The Endocrine System

The base chakra is located at the base of your spine and corresponds to your adrenal gland which is responsible for the production of adrenalin. Being close to the anus it relates to matter (e.g. fecal matter), food and other basic needs.

The sacral chakra is located in your pelvis and corresponds to the gonads (testicles or ovaries). It is connected with sexual energy and relationships.

The solar plexus chakra is located in your tummy region and corresponds to the pancreas which controls digestion, regulates blood sugar and produces enzymes. It's also linked to your 'gut' feelings.

The heart chakra is located in your chest and corresponds to the thymus gland which is responsible for your immune system. It is associated with feelings of love and belonging.

The throat chakra is located in your throat and corresponds to your thyroid gland which regulates your metabolic rate. It is associated with our ability to express, also relates intellectual thinking, which is expressed through our words.

The third eye chakra is situated in the space between your eyebrows, near your brain's neo-cortex, and corresponds to the pituitary gland which regulates hormone secretion. This is linked to spiritual and psychic thought.

Finally your crown chakra is at the top of your head and corresponds to your hypothalamus which regulates sleep and hunger. Being above and beyond your brain, it is linked to spiritual transcendence.

Getting To The Root Of The Matter

The two lower chakras are located within the moving centre. Your root chakra is located in the hip area at the base of your spine. This chakra relates to your primal material and survival needs. If you have money issues, or you are overly concerned about your material needs, this can often relate to a blocked root chakra. A healthy root chakra energy represents an ability to stand up for and support yourself in your life. You will have a sense of independence and self sufficiency. Where the energy in this area is blocked, emotions include: fear, envy, shame, loneliness and depression. Physical symptoms will include: lower back pain, sciatica, varicose veins, bowel disorders and immune related disorders.

Your sacral chakra is located within your sexual organs and is the seat of your emotions. This chakra is the storage centre for all your experiences associated with love and hate. The feelings of acceptance or rejection from yourself and others influence the relationships created in your life.

The sacral chakra also influences how you express your emotions. It relates to how you relate to other people, your tribe (family), authority and being able to feel in control of your personal needs. A balanced sacral chakra helps you to express your emotions without being too emotional, and opens you to passion, intimacy and sexuality.

As mentioned before, this area also contains your sexual energy, which is about your ability to fully trust and be open to intimacy in your personal relationships. A past hurt can cause a withdrawal of your energy in this area. If you 'cover up' your feelings to do with sexuality and intimacy, then this may result in layers of excess fat over your hips and bottom. This chakra also influences how well you're able to express your creativity. Symptoms of a blocked sacral chakra include: hormone imbalances, infertility, cystitis, money and sexual problems, dependency and handing your power over, blame and guilt.

Exercise #10:
Do The Hippy Hippy Shake

Here are a couple of exercises to loosen up your hips and buttocks to get your energy in this area activated and flowing. Exercising and loosening your hips and buttocks will help you to shift any unhealthy mindset attached to this area. Connecting to any resistance you experience, is the key to uncovering any underlying issues.

Stand in a comfortable position with your legs about a foot apart. Keep your knees soft and tilt your pelvis backwards and forwards. Move only your pelvis and not your upper body or legs. Notice how much movement you have here. Are they loose or tight?

Now swing your hips from side to side by bending one knee and allowing your opposite hip to drop to the other side. Check that your upper body and your legs stay upright.

How far do your hips move? Are they flexible or inflexible? Now rotate your hips as if you were a belly dancer or using a hoola hoop, making sure your upper body isn't moving. Is this easy for you? Is the energy flowing freely in your hips? Is there any discomfort or resistance?

If so, what words describe what it feels like. What do you think this represents? Write your answers down.

Exercising Your Soul Muscles

This is a great and simple exercise to help open up your hips especially the very important psoas muscle which runs internally from your lower back to the top of your legs. In ancient Chinese tradition, the psoas is known as the seat of the muscle of the soul. Lay on your back with your knees bent and your feet are on the floor about two feet apart.

Move your left knee in towards your body to the space on the floor between your legs, your left foot should be out to your side. Now move that same leg into the opposite direction so that your knee is out and your foot is beside the inside of your right thigh.

Repeat this movement 8 times, bringing your knee in and out. Bring your awareness to all the muscles you are using, particularly in your spine and hip. When you have finished, notice the difference in your left hip to your right hip. Does it feel freer? Looser? More open? Can you feel the energy in your left side tingling and moving?

Now swap your legs and do it to the other side. Notice if any words or emotions come to you.

If this exercise is difficult, listen to the quality of the feelings behind any physical discomfort you experience. Was there any tightness or discomfort? What was the feeling behind the discomfort? Write down your word or phrase.

The Tale Of The Frustrated Dancer

When one of my clients, Layla, tried this exercise for the first time all she kept saying was, it's stuck, it doesn't want to move'.

I asked her what this stuckness felt like. She said, 'it feels like it's trapped and can't get free'.

So I asked her how this felt. "Suffocating," she replied, 'I feel frustrated. I want it to be free but it won't go'.

I asked her how this related to her sense of independence, her direction in life and her creativity. She thought about it for a bit, then she nodded knowingly. It turns out she used to be a dancer and longed to dance again, but her husband didn't want her to. He was frightened that if she started to dance again, then she'd find new friends and a new freedom and would then want to leave him. She had allowed him to make the decisions and allowed herself to be disempowered. She used his reasoning as an excuse not to follow her heart and had accepted that this was how it was meant to be. Her body however believed otherwise and realising this empowered Layla to make changes in her relationship and take a new direction in life, training as a dance teacher.

Now you have got to know your hips and buttocks better, write down what you think your hips and buttocks say about you regarding your direction in life? Do you experience ease and flow in this area or is there a resistance? How easy it is for you to be spontaneous and to surrender to change? How easy is it to express yourself emotionally and sexually?

What can you start to do differently to bring the energy in this area into healthy balance, by changing your posture and/or thinking patterns?

♥ Meditation #3:
Footprints In The Sand

During this next guided meditation, you will get a better under-standing of the messages or thoughts your are holding onto in your moving centre. Give yourself this opportunity to tune in a little deeper to your unconscious and listen to the MindBody messages hidden in your hips and buttocks.

This meditation will help you to transform the old programming and create new, healthier thought patterns. The more you repeat the meditations the greater the results. Read through it first or get someone to read it out to you. You will need to allow at least 20 minutes for this exercise.

Lay or sit in a comfortable position and take a couple of deep breaths until your body is relaxed. Bring your entire moving centre (your hips, legs and knees and feet) to your awareness and listen to the feelings or words that come up? Is there a key word that you repeatedly used during your exercises?

Does this word relate to any problems, emotions or issues attached to this area in the past? They could be sexual issues; giving birth or not giving birth; fertility issues or unhealthy relationships. What are you holding onto emotionally in this area? Did you abort any creative ideas that you once had but didn't follow through on? Do you have any fears related to your own financial security or future security?

Allow any thoughts or feelings to arise. Just listen to your thoughts and feelings without judgment, just acknowledge them and allow these feelings to expand. Welcome the feelings. Allow the feelings to grow bigger so they can be fully expressed. Feel all emotions and fears attached to these though patterns. You are safe to express these feelings however you want to.

Now Imagine this feeling as a shape or colour within the centre of your pelvis. It might look like grey ball or black treacle. This is trapped or stuck energy which is from your past and which no longer serves you or needs to be there. Observe the shape without judgment. Now Imagine the shape dissolving into nothing, bit by bit it disappears until it is no longer there. Take your time. Breathe it out until it has gone. Notice any resistance to letting it go.

Now imagine you are under a waterfall of pure water and picture the water cascading down your spine washing and cleansing the hip area. Washing it all clean away.

There is now a warm red ball of glowing light, like the setting sun, glowing in the space within your pelvis. Imagine this warm glowing light is filled with love for you. Feel it grow bigger and bigger, brighter and brighter. Feel it glowing brightly and growing until it feels so big and bright that it radiates throughout your whole body. Feel your whole being radiating with this warm red glow. Feel its warm loving support as it recharges your whole pelvic region.

Now imagine this red light getting smaller and smaller again until it is the size of a tennis ball sitting between your hips, glowing, warming, healing and full of loving energy to move you forward. This is your base chakra, which is now healthy and rich with new life. You can now go forward with no restrictions or blocks. You are free. You are now ready to step into life ready to truly walk your talk.

Take a deep breath in and slowly open your eyes. Make sure you allow time to fully return to awareness before you go about your normal activities.

+

The final exercise in this chapter is to create your positive affirmation or statement, using the words you wrote as a guide to know what you need to change. Repeat this affirmation every day or as often as you feel you need to.

My affirmation to reprogram the language of my hips and buttocks is:..

....

KEY LESSONS FROM CHAPTER EIGHT

- **Become more aware of your hips, they will tell you how free you truly feel to move through all areas of your life, however you want to**

CHAPTER NINE

Your Being Centre

In this chapter we're going to explore your 'being centre'. Take a moment to set your intention for this section of Your Mind-Body journey as you prepare to focus on the human experience we call 'being'.

Your 'being centre', is located in the upper portion of your body. This centre represents how you are 'being' in your life. It relates to socialising, communicating and expressing yourself. Firstly lets focus on the back of your being centre, this is your spine and your central nervous system (CNS).

The spine is your life support system. It is the place that holds you together. The muscles supporting your spine are what shapes you physically, mentally and emotionally. It is where the CNS runs (your main nerve channel). It is the backbone of your life and all your personal responsibilities. It is your own personal support network and relates to your core strength, your will power, your self esteem and your 'backbone'.

If you are feeling unsupported in life it will show up as weakness in your back. The back represents the unconscious where we dump issues that we don't want to deal with. Thoughts like 'I'm not being supported' or 'I'm being let down' can translate into back pain or weakness. We can stand up for ourselves and walk tall or bow down with the weight of the world's problems on our shoulders, as we 'bend over backwards' and 'shoulder the burden' or our own and other peoples' expectations.

The lower back represents the weight and responsibility of being human, money worries and our sense of security. The physical support we need to take care of the basic practicalities of life. If you have lower back problems, ask yourself if you are getting the physical support you need? If you have lower back pain you will probably find that your abdominal muscles are weak, as your spine is doing more than its fair share of work supporting you.

Your mid-back holds the balance in the centre of the body, it represents your decision making processes and the balance you strike between your own needs and demands of others. It can be the place in the body where you hold onto guilt and a lack of self forgiveness. It also relates to feeling emotionally unsupported. Are you getting your emotional needs met in the way that works for you, or do you carry the weight of supporting others emotionally?

The upper back muscles hold onto anger. If you hold onto anger from the past that has not been expressed and healed, then it can transform into spite and bitterness and become trapped in your MindBody and control all your actions, motives and expressions. Do you have, or have you had, back issues in the past? Do you, or did you, feel a lack of support financially, emotionally or physically?

If you have issues with your back in general, are you being spineless? Are you overwhelmed by responsibility for others and bending over backwards? Or are you holding back? Do you feel like you are going backwards? Or are you turning your back on something you don't want to face?

The Tale of One Woman Who Went To Mow

Sarah's husband had recently left her. She was hurt, resentful and angry. She was striding towards the shed where the lawn mower was kept, seething and cursing that she had to cut the lawn, as this used to be one of her husband's duties.

Even before she picked up the mower, her back went into spasm and then her whole back seized up. She could barely walk let alone mow the lawn! So she came to see me so that I could do remedial massage work on her back.

As she told this story I asked her what she was thinking just before her back went out. She said, 'I was cursing my ex-husband for landing me with all the responsibilities, particularly the finances and lawn mowing, all the things men are 'meant' to do!'. Sarah was avoiding being responsible for herself. She always relied on her husband to do the things she didn't want to do. Years later, after taking more responsibility for her life, she came to realise that her husband leaving her was a blessing, she became more 'whole' and complete. Her masculine and feminine energies became balanced, she found her 'backbone' and for her, there was now no turning back!

Problems in any area of the body are often linked to the spine because your centre of gravity is not in balance, because some of your muscles in one area of your body are either too tight or too weak. These imbalances often start with you feeling emotionally out of balance. Your feelings are created by your thoughts and your thoughts manifest in your body and also in your life.

Retraining muscles to work in balance starts with re-training your mind. This unlocks the sensory motor amnesia (muscles that have gone to sleep due to accidents, injury or trauma and that have been programmed not to work). If you cannot sense a muscle, you cannot move it. The more you can sense a muscle the more you can move it, enabling the muscles to work within their 'muscle group' effectively.

If you have noticed that your posture has got into bad habits over time, that your shoulders may be hunched, or your spine is curved, then what thoughts do you think you are habitually having to create this? What does your back and spine say about you, particularly regarding your ability or need to support yourself?

Exercise #11:
Developing Your Backbone

Here are some physical exercises to stretch and loosen the muscles, which in turn will help to release the blocks and stored memory in this area. They also help to strengthen and re-shape your spine to help embody a feeling of being able to support yourself. These exercises are particularly good for bad backs and correcting green light and red light postures. While you are doing these exercises, notice any resistance or feelings of discomfort, and be open to new insights about what this may mean to you.

Lay on the floor facing downwards with your arms stretched out in front of you and your legs open. You look like a big 'X'. Bring your chin on to the floor so that your spine is straight. Lift your opposite arm and leg with the in breath and bring it back down with the out breath (alternating your right leg with left arm, then left leg and right arm). Swap sides. Do this ten times. Notice if one side of the body is less flexible or weaker than the other.

Now place your body on to all fours with your knees on the floor and your hands directly under your shoulders with your arms straight. This is the classic cat position. This stretch is brilliant to increase the flexibility of the spine, loosening the vertebrae, keeping the CNS healthy and to ease lower back pain. In fact if you did this exercise every day, you would reduce the chances of suffering back pain ever again! Breathe in and raise your head towards the ceiling and tilt your pelvis outward sagging your belly towards the floor. Breathe out and curl your spine up towards the ceiling, head and buttocks curling under. Squeeze your core muscles at the end of your out breath. And again, breathe in, head up, tailbone up with belly sagging and then again breathe out and curl under. Repeat this back and forth action with the in and out breath ten times.

Next you will retrain your posture by using neuromuscular (MindBody) training which will not only retrain your body but will also rewire your mindset attached.

Biofeedback Neuromuscular Training

Do you remember the exercise you did in Chapter 6 to feel centred and balanced? This is where you were standing with the weight in your feet distributed evenly on the floor, your spine was straight, your shoulders were rolled back and your head sitting comfortably at the top of your spine. You were centred in your hara. In yoga practice we call this Tadasana or Mountain Pose.

Stand facing a full-length mirror if you have one, or a partner if not. Observe your posture in the mirror or get your partner to tell you if your body is in a straight line. You may find one shoulder is dropped on one side, or your spine is slightly bent to one side, or your head may be slightly tilted, or one of your hip bones is higher than the other.

Be observant, see how your spine has adapted over time to become the shape it is. Using the mirror or your partner to help you, lengthen your spine by thinking tall, straighten your body so that your shoulders are level and not rolling forward, your ears are directly above your shoulders. Check that your pelvis is not tilted to one side and you're neither in green light or red light posture, but somewhere in-between.

This new way of standing might feel very strange and unnatural at first and your body will want to default back to its usual posture. This is quite normal as the body assumes the old way of holding your body is the 'correct' way, after years of programming. To retrain your posture so that it naturally defaults into Mountain Pose and to a healthier spine shape, we will now practice biofeedback training.

Once you are in Mountain Pose, close your eyes and sense how this new posture feels. Hold onto this feeling until your memory retains it. Now lean to one side, then to the other, then forward, then backward, then back to the centre. Before you open your eyes again, sense your way back to the corrected posture. Your body will want to automatically go back to its usual spine shape, but this is where the training comes in. The more you can 'sense' your way back to the new posture, rather than looking to correct it, the more you'll find you can adapt quite quickly to your new posture.

Once you have sensed your way back to your corrected posture, open your eyes and check it is still straight. If it isn't and it has gone back to the old posture, then close your eyes again, lean forward and back then side to side, then again sense your way back to Mountain Pose. Keep doing this until your partner or the mirror confirms your posture is straight. If you practice this on a regular basis until you no longer have to sense your way back to your new posture, then your neuromuscular feedback training is complete. This is the type of exercise you can practice in lots of different places, in the kitchen, in the supermarket queue, when you're stuck at a social event being bored by someone you're not really listening to!

The more you practice, the sooner you'll find you can automatically default to your new way of holding your body.

During these exercises, were there any feelings of discomfort, resistance or inflexibility in your back? If so, what do you think this represents in terms of your feelings about being supported and taking responsibility?

If there was discomfort, resistance or inflexibility, what was the feeling behind the discomfort? Use a word or phrase to describe this and write down your answers.

How do you think you can change your posture and your thoughts patterns to create a healthy spine and CNS?

Write a positive affirmation or statement, using the words you've noted down as a guide and repeat this affirmation every day or as often as you can remember. Saying your affirmation with feeling instead of just thinking your affirmation will help you create you new programming.

It is important that you use your affirmation in the present tense. For example; 'I am supported where all my needs are met'. Also remember that if you use a negative as your affirmation, for example; 'I no longer feel pain', your subconscious only responds to the words and thoughts you use and so will only hear the word 'pain'. Therefore you will more than likely experience more pain.

My affirmation to reprogram the language of my spine is:

....

....

The Art Of Being Zen

Now let's focus on the front part of your being centre, this is your abdomen, solar plexus and your chest. This area of your body represents your conscious self.

Together, your torso and your hara is your personal energy engine. It is where you hold your confidence, self-esteem, self-acceptance and your intuition. All of your daily activities radiate from your hara, your lower belly. Most westerners however, have their centre of being focused in the busyness of their heads, which is more ego based.

By centring yourself from your abdomen, your body's centre of gravity, you can begin to develop a more 'zen' way being. This means being both powerful but relaxed, to have self confidence without ego, to be present in your actions and to have MindBody awareness in all you do.

This area is very vulnerable as it contains all of your internal organs. Your limbic brain has an inherent need to protect it from things that could bring it danger. This is why you might subconsciously turn slightly to the side when someone you dislike approaches you. This centre is where you store your 'gut' feelings and your intuitions. This is where you feel your inner most emotions.

Energy In Motion = Emotion

Our emotions grow out of our guts. Your feelings need a path-way for expression, as your legs express your direction and your arms express your actions, your emotions need an avenue to be expressed too. If you don't express your feelings, then these blocked emotions can create a dam, a block in your energy which can explode into anger, or fester as sorrow or depression, stress, stiff muscles, stomach ulcers etc. Maybe you have been taught as a child to not fully express yourself and so you now act out how you are supposed to feel as opposed to how you really feel. Your conditioned mind controls your feelings. It is therefore important to get to know what's really going on inside of you to prevent blocked energy.

Do any of the descriptions below relate to you?

Large Extended Bellies: this relates to unexpressed creativity causing your energy to be stuck.

Fat Bellies: relates to covering up your sensitivities, emotions and low self esteem with protection.

Solar Plexus: Your tummy region is where your solar plexus chakra is located. This is where your personal power and self-esteem is filtered. It is where you pick up on your 'gut' feelings. It is your inner compass from where you are nudged and guided forward by your inner knowing. It is where your 'chi' power, what is known in Eastern traditions, flows.

Illness or heath issues around the abdomen are activated by low self-esteem, lack of self-responsibility, fears of not being good enough, fear of rejection and over sensitivity to criticism. You can usually use any stomach problems as a barometer of your emotional state.

Do you use language like, 'I can't stomach it', or 'I feel gutted' or, 'this is hard to digest', 'I'm sick of it'. 'I feel sick to the stomach'. 'I haven't got the guts'?

You can usually tell what type of character you are by what your internal organs are doing. Your tummy will feel tight when you are in stressful situations, or you could be holding on to unresolved emotions and blocked feelings which might lead to tummy upsets, and digestion problems.

Or if you have trained yourself not to express 'hard' feelings, then you may overcompensate by displaying a gentle and fragile personality and will seldom engage in assertive, forceful or aggressive actions. You literally can't stomach it, which can result in having butterflies in your stomach, tummy ulcers, indigestion or irritable bowel syndrome. If your emotional energy is locked up like a caged animal desperate for release, then it will cause havoc internally.

The Tale Of The Women Who Ate Herself

One of my clients, Katrina, suffered badly from indigestion for years. No matter what she ate she still had indigestion. Day and night it persisted. She tried everything to get to the bottom of it, fasting, dieting, homeopathy, kinesiology, massage, herbal remedies, digestive enzymes, aloe vera. You name it, she tried it and still her indigestion was bad.

I asked her what it was that she couldn't stomach. She then told me the story of her ongoing family upset. She had been betrayed badly by a couple of family members and she felt sad that she had been betrayed by the people she loved and trusted the most.

It was literally eating away at her. I gave her body an energy healing and when I got to the area on her back, directly over her stomach, I felt a void of energy and the overwhelming pain of her feelings of her betrayal.

She had energetically and literally been stabbed in the back!! We reclaimed that energy loss and I helped her to let go and forgive the people who were 'eating away at her insides'.

The next day she phoned me full of joy. She said, 'I can't believe this but my indigestion has completely gone! I cannot thank you enough'. This is why I love my work!

Your personal power is held within your solar plexus. This is different to your will power. Will power is a determined force, which is useful when overpowering the ego. Personal power is a passive power, which I know sounds contradictory.

Personal power is a state of being not a state of doing. It is an inner confidence, a knowing and a trust in yourself and the choices you make in life. It is your courage to step forward and be the person you were born to be. It is a self-confidence and assurance without the presence of arrogance or ego.

Personal power is gained with the growth of your self-esteem and to develop your self-esteem, you sometimes need to strengthen it by facing challenges. If your self-esteem is low, then here are some important questions to ask yourself.

What is it about myself that I don't like or accept? What false belief have I made up about who I am that runs my life? Do I make choices in life from love or from fear? Do I make choices in life that strengthen me or weaken me? Do I choose to have friends that strengthen me or weaken me? What do I allow in my life that makes me feel weak or takes my personal power away? Do I accept who I am regardless of my 'faults'? What do your answers say about your personal power?

If you feel disempowered most of the time (which is feeling like you are not in control of your life and that others or 'life' seems to make all the decisions for you) then perhaps you have an unhealthy programming regarding what you associate with the word 'power'.

So how can you reclaim your personal power? In the next chapter we'll look more closely at the lower front section of your 'being centre' where your personal power is held.

KEY LESSONS FROM CHAPTER NINE

- **Your spine is your life support system, by being aware of and learning to adjust your posture will transform your feelings of support, self-esteem and your ability to take responsibility for your life**

CHAPTER TEN

Your Power

In this chapter we're going to explore your personal power. Be sure to set your intention for this chapter as it is designed to ignite the 'fire in your belly'!

What do you associate with the word power? Is it strength? Force? Domination and control? Men? Something else?

If you have a negative or unhealthy association with the word power, then you're certainly not going to want to become empowered yourself! If you associate power with force, then you will become passive. If you associate power with physical strength being used for harm, then you'll become weak. If you associate power with control, then you'll become unruly and undisciplined. If you're a woman who associates power with men, then you may disown the masculine energy within you.

Your true power is the mastery over how you think, believe, feel and respond to life. It is about being able to create whatever you want in your life, no matter what your circumstances. Your thoughts create your life and therefore whatever you think, will shape your everyday experiences. You will have challenges throughout your life, yet it isn't the experience that most impacts you, rather it is how you react to or interpret those experiences that has the biggest effect.

Fears are not real, they are just your thought projections. The emotions you feel are not real as they are created through your mind from past experiences and your programming.

The more you operate from your centre, then the less the external ups and downs of life will affect you. And the more you learn to operate from your centre, your hara, as opposed to your mind, your emotions or your programming, then the more secure you will become with who you really are and your true self.

Choose It Or Change It?

Do you sometimes struggle with staying in your power, your centre and your truth? Do you believe you don't have the power to change certain circumstances in your life? Then I say you have three choices. You can choose it, you can change it, or you can walk away. When you make one of these choices to something that troubles you in life, then you will reclaim your power.

I love the serenity prayer: 'God, give us the serenity to accept what cannot be changed, the courage to change what can be changed and the wisdom to know the difference.'

In my MindBody Journey Course we do a group exercise that demonstrates just how powerful we all are. I ask a volunteer to sit on a chair, then I ask four people in the group to stand by this person. Two people stand behind facing this person's back, the other two are beside them. Then I ask the four people who are standing to place their hands into a yoga position called 'steeple mudra', by interlacing their fingers and releasing the index fingers to form a point.

Next, I ask the four people standing to slip their pointed index fingers under the person sitting. The two people behind place their fingers under the sitter's armpits and the two people at the side under their bended knees. Then I ask them to lift the seated person off the chair. Of course they can't do it, even a light person is impossible to lift up using just the index fingers.

But then I ask the four people who are standing to do it again. This time they get themselves into their centres, focus all their attention on their breath and direct the breath downwards. This helps to anchor them. I make sure they all have their focus on their inner power, their hara, then I count them down...

Five, Four, Three, Two, One... They all breathe in and on the count of 'one' they slide their index fingers back under the sitting person's body and they lift them up into the air. This time the seated person seems to be as light as a feather and they can lift them easily, sometimes right up to the ceiling! This demonstration works every single time I do it and has always worked no matter how heavy the seated person is. I have used men and women and the result is always the same. However, I have learnt to be watchful of people's reactions, because on the first occasion I tried it with a group, the four lifters were so shocked when their volunteer almost touched the ceiling that they dropped them to the floor! It's okay, no damage was done, just lots of hysterical laughing.

I use this demonstration as it was something that used to be done as a party trick with a bit of 'mumbo jumbo' thrown in for good measure to make people think that it's magic. I am now going to be a spoilsport and tell you the secret of how it's done! I do this because I believe everyone deserves the right to know about their own power.

There are four key factors, or 'pillars of power', that need to be in place simultaneously. They are **Attention** (focus), **Intention, Action** and **Trust**. These are the ingredients for manifestation and can be applied to anything. We have all heard of examples of miraculous stories such as a child running into the road, getting run over by a car and the mother lifting the car to retrieve their child from under it. Or a karate expert who breaks concrete in half with his bare hands.

This power is there for all of us to use at any time, and not just for lifting heavy objects. It is there for us to use to manifest all that we deserve, yet most of us never use it. Instead we focus on our limitations and beliefs about how something can't work.

It is usually only through challenging life experiences that most people experience themselves drawing upon this power so they can miraculously pull through.

Of course we don't even have to wait until we have a major life crisis before we call upon our power, we can use it in any day to day scenarios.

The Tale Of The Amazing Walking Woman

I was struggling up a rather steep hill one day on one of my walks, huffing and puffing and not at all enjoying it. I stopped and gave myself a good talking to. For goodness

sake, I am a fit woman and I have the tools to stop the struggle, but sometimes I forget to use them. So I focused on my intention (to get to the top of the hill), breathed in to my belly and my chi power, told myself that climbing the hill is effortless and off I went.

I was breathing into my core and before I knew it I was at the top! It was so easy, what was all the fuss about? I even stormed past a man who was jogging on the way and he shook his head with disbelief as I overtook him. "Something's not quite right," he said "I think it's time I gave up! How come you can walk faster than I can run?"

Exercise #12:
Building Your Core Strength

Can you think of any situations in your past when you found you had the strength, physically or emotionally when you believed you had none? Use the following core strengthening exercises to practice your inner power, by utilising the four 'pillars of power': Attention, Intention, Action and Trust.

Lay on the floor facing upwards with your knees bent. Breathe in and with the out breath, push your lower back into the floor and hold. Breathe normally but keep your lower spine pressed against the floor. Soon you will be able to feel your inner core muscles engage. This is a useful and safe exercise to try if you have back problems.

To advance this exercise, interlace your fingers and bring them to behind your head. Keeping your knees bent and your feet on the floor hip width apart. Take a deep breath in and on your out breath bring your head off the floor keeping your shoulders and neck soft. Hold for as long as you feel comfortable to do so. This will tone up all your abdominal muscles, helping to strengthen your spine. Remember to keep breathing while you hold.

Listen to the thoughts that swim around your head during these exercises. What are these thoughts saying to you?

Do these thoughts belong to a familiar pattern of thinking that shows up when things start to get tough in your life?

To advance the exercise to another level, with your back on the floor, breathe in again and on the out breath come all the way up into a sit up. Were you able to do this easily? If so, your core muscles are strong. If you didn't then we will now practice it again, but this time using your chi power! Make sure you use the right thoughts or words while you do this exercise, choosing strong, simple statements like 'I Will!' Remember your intention here is to fully sit up and remember your power. Breathe fully into your belly and with the out breath direct your breath down towards your toes and sit up. Make your breath loud as you exhale, like a karate master. Was it easier this time?

If you had a problem with breathing out loudly, then why did you? Are you afraid of expressing and showing your power?

During these core strengthening exercises was there any discomfort or resistance or weakness in your tummy? If so, what do you think this represents for you?

What was the feeling behind the discomfort? Use a word or phrase. What negative words or phrases were trying to sabotage this exercise for you?

Here are some questions to help you:

● Do you lack inner power or self esteem?
● Do you believe in who you are and how you are being?
● Do you have good self-esteem, self-confidence, self-respect and self-honour?
● Do you have will power? Are you confident in your decisions?
● Are you sensitive to criticism?
● Tune into the tummy area and ask what it's REALLY feeling.
● What is it that you are hiding in there?

What can you change to bring your core being, your personal power back to health?

Write down anything that will help you change your posture and/or your thinking patterns?

Write your affirmation or statement (for example 'I love to express my power and passion'). Repeat this affirmation with feeling as often as you can as it will help retrain your neural pathways.

My affirmation to reprogram the language of my stomach is: ....

....

♥ Meditation #4: Finding Your Inner Power

Find yourself into a quiet space and allow yourself ten minutes to do this simple meditation that will help you develop your self-esteem and personal power. Read it through first or get someone to read it to you.

Breathe deeply and allow your body to soften and relax. Ask yourself if there are any feelings from the past that you are still holding onto? Unfulfilled dreams? Regrets?

Now imagine yourself being the person that you would like yourself to be. Would you be more confident, more loved or loving, more open, more assertive, fitter, calmer? Whatever it is that you deeply desire for yourself imagine what that would be like. You can change anything in your life just by changing how you think and feel.

Now Imagine that you are that person. Imagine how you would walk, talk and be in any situation. See this person in your mind's eye fully and deeply. If you have problems with visualising then just feel what you would feel like. Embrace the feeling in every nerve and cell of your being. Be this person.

This person in your imagination is you. It is the you without any blocks, fears, hurts, upsets or lack of self-esteem. This person is within you waiting to be expressed. It has always been you and will always be you. You are this person when you are in your power. Stay for as long as you need to in this feeling space, embodying and engraving your true essence deep into your MindBody.

Be it. Breathe it. Live it.

You are it.

Now take that person with you into the next week and beyond. Open your eyes and notice how different you and your body feels. You have generated these feelings just by your thoughts. You can do this all the time. It's up to you.

KEY LESSONS FROM CHAPTER TEN

- **Tune into your gut on a daily basis and learn to access your personal power, and know that you can achieve whatever you want in life**

CHAPTER ELEVEN

Your Chest

The final area of your 'being centre' we'll be exploring is your chest. Be sure to set a positive intention and prepare to approach this chapter with an open heart.

Your chest is the area where you hold your self-identity, it is your direct relationship to your self. It is the 'I' when you point to your chest indicating your identity. It is where you hold your pride or where you put on a good front. It is where you hold your feelings about yourself, your self love and your humility.

Is your chest open and full of pride or is it an area that you protect, holding things close to your chest, protecting your heart? The breast is where we, as humans, provide nourishment for our young, whether that's a mother breastfeeding her baby or the father's breast swelling with pride as he feeds and nurtures his child, with words of praise and encouragement.

Most obviously our chest plays home to our lungs, which breathe us into life on an ongoing, daily basis. On average, most people only use about 30 percent of their lung capacity and most of us breathe only into our upper chest (the thorax). Often we don't breathe fully into our diaphragm and into the lower chambers of our lungs.

Research into cardiac patients who suffered heart attacks or aneurysms has found that they tend to be thoracic breathers and not diaphragmatic breathers. If you are a shallow breather, it will increase your heart beat and the faster your heart beats then the higher your blood pressure will be.

Shallow breathing sets off our fight/flight/freeze hormones, making us think we are in danger and because our body thinks we are in danger, then our heart rate increases. It is a vicious circle of stress. When we're in constant stress, anxiety or fear, it limits our breathing, cutting us off from our natural life force.

How can we fully live and feel when we are effectively holding our breath by not using our lungs full capacity? Put another way, how can we hope to live life to the full when we don't use our lungs to their fullest potential?

If you have problems with breathing, it may be because you have forgotten how to breathe correctly. If your posture is more of a red light posture, for example, then you are more than likely to be a shallow breather.

Exercise #13:
Getting To Know Your Lungs

The following exercise will help you to optimise the use of your lungs. You can do this exercise standing up or sitting down, whatever is most comfortable for you.

Thoracic breathing: firstly take a few small shallow breaths into the top part of your chest keeping your tummy muscles tight. How does it make you feel? Anxious? Stressed? Tense? Alert? Now breathe a long breath out. How did that make you feel? Relaxed? Relieved? Your blood pressure automatically decreases on the out breath and increases again on the in breath.

Diaphragmatic breathing: now breathe deeply in and out from your belly long slow deep breaths. Count to six as you inhale and then exhale to the count of eight. On your in-breath your tummy should swell and finally the air filters into the top of your chest. On your exhale the opposite happens, the air goes out from your chest first, the sides of your ribs draw inwards and your belly flattens. It might take practice if you're used to breathing from your chest only.

After a few breaths of diaphragmatic breathing allow your breath to get back to its normal rhythm. How do you feel now? Relaxed? Calm? If you feel yourself getting giddy, you are probably still breathing from your upper chest.

A simple way to practice diaphragmatic breathing if you are new to this is to lay on your back with your knees bent and your feet on the floor. Breathe in swelling the belly and tilting your pelvis out, arching the back, then breathe out pushing your spine into the floor and your pelvis tilting under. Repeat this several times.

Lateral breathing: this is the best breath to use on a daily basis as your normal breathing rhythm. When you practice lateral breathing, you breathe into the sides of your ribs only, so that your ribs fan out to their sides and then draw back into your chest. The action is like the bellows used to stoke an old fashioned fire. This way of breathing encourages your breath to travel downwards into the bottom of your lungs, as opposed to staying in the top of your chest. Spend some time today tuning into how you breathe and catch yourself out.

You may be surprised at how much you hold your breath.

If you have regular chest problems, chest infections or coughs then it could be due to you holding onto emotions or protecting yourself from facing your feelings. Are you wanting to get something off your chest? Do you hold your feelings close to your chest? Are you holding your breath in order to keep life on hold? Do you love yourself and treat yourself with kindness and nurturing thoughts and deeds?

The Tale Of The Bag Lady Who Faced Her Fears

Beverley came to me because of a persistent sore neck, which had troubled her for years, despite regular treatments by an osteopath. She also suffered from quite severe asthma, which would flare up when she was stressed. In addition, she had low self-esteem and her familiar pattern in life was that others would treat her disrespectfully.

The root cause was that she didn't and couldn't love herself. She was worried that if she looked inside herself, she wouldn't like what she found. She built up a fear which grew bigger and bigger. This was mirrored in her size and body fat, wrapping around her for protection. She had put the lid on her emotions, which would get to boiling point, rising up to her neck, then eventually erupting as either asthma or a full-blown panic attack.

In my first session with Beverley, we unraveled her negative thought patterns and programming and discovered that this had developed as a result of a poor relationship with her father. Then in our next session together, we looked at her inner child and how hurt and misunderstood it still felt. I encouraged Beverley to work at loving the inner child using a meditation in which she sent love to the little girl inside her through a mirror, reflecting the love back at her. This indirect way of giving love to herself helped work around her resistance to loving herself directly.

I also did some energy healing work. During this healing, an affirmation was given to her by her inner voice. This was, 'no more fear, only love'. She went out of the session repeating her mantra again and again, passionately and with emotion.

By the third session she arrived for her treatment full of beans, as she had finally begun to face her fears. It turned out that Beverley's mother died 15 years earlier and she had been given a bag of her mother's belongings, which she immediately shoved in her loft without looking inside. She was so scared of facing her emotions when opening this bag, she'd even tightly wrapped the bag up in sheets and blankets.

Beverley was scared that if she looked inside the bag she wouldn't like what she found---just as she was scared that if she dared to look within, she wouldn't like what she found. The thoughts she was thinking about herself, that had manifested in her body, were also showing up in her life. She wrapped the bag in blankets---just like she had wrapped herself in metaphorical cotton wool---to try and prevent herself from getting hurt.

After session two, with the help of her new mantra, 'no more fear, only love', she bravely climbed into the loft, removed the dusty material that had been wrapped around her mother's bag for over a decade and found the courage to look inside.

Inside she discovered a few bits of nice jewellery, some documents and a wad of cash worth £500! So instead of finding things she wouldn't like she found the exact opposite. She found wealth and beauty. She realised this was symbolic of the fact that if she dared to look inside herself, she would find the same.

So by session three she had shocked herself by doing two things which were out of character for her. She took a long trip on a train to confront a friend who had treated her badly many years ago and told her how she felt. This helped her feel empowered, liberated and self-confident. She also started to believe she was worthy of love and expressed that by buying herself some new clothes and had a new hair cut.

Three months later, Beverley's asthma had gone, she had changed her job and she was happier than she had ever been. She had come to peace with her father and her troubled childhood and her neck pain had also disappeared, because the 'pain in the neck' in her life and the ability to assert herself by 'doing' something about it, had now been resolved.

Open Up Your Heart Chakra

Your chest is where your heart chakra lives. When the heart is engaged, it drives your body to act on your mind's ideas. When your heart energy is absent, when 'your heart is not in it', your actions have no power. When your mind and heart are congruent, that is, when your heart and mind are in alignment, you act confidently, fearlessly and make good choices.

Your heart chakra is connected to your thymus gland, which corresponds with your immune system, so when you experience loving positive feelings your immune system is strong. When your heart chakra is not open, when you are not loving, but feel fearful or negative emotions, the thymus gland will weaken, which in turn weakens your immune system.

Loving yourself will heal you. Love stimulates your immune system and your white blood cells. Your heart chakra is an extremely powerful energetic centre. When you express your love, your compassion and your emotions, the energy from this transmits outwards.

There have been many experiments to test the power of our heart energy, particularly with remote healing. Remote healing is where someone sends love and healing for another through their heart and consciously directing it to the subject of their intention. Remarkable miracles of healing have occurred that no one can explain. This is the true power of love.

One example of the power of love in action, is the story a new baby girl born prematurely with most of her organs not functioning. She was wired up to life support machines but the doctors didn't have much hope for her and she was showing signs of deterioration. Eventually there was nothing more the doctors could do and the machines were turned off.

The mother and father of this new born baby refused to believe that their little baby girl was going to leave them so soon. They took it in turns to hold the babe in their arms and for five days and five nights they poured pure love and devotion into this baby. They even asked their friends and relatives to pray for their little girl, which they did. On the sixth day the baby's heart beat was strong and all her internal organs were functioning normally. The doctors were baffled. Reading this story in the media touched my heart and reminded me of the power of our heart centre. Love heals.

Physically, what does your chest say about you? Are you protecting your heart with your shoulders rounded? Do you regularly fold your arms over your chest? Do you naturally breathe deeply into your belly with your chest open? And are you a calm, centred person? Or do you mainly breathe from your chest and in stress mode a lot of the time? What does this say about you emotionally? What is your heart really saying to you? If you had a broken heart from the past, what resentments or hurts is your heart still holding onto?

The Power Of Forgiveness

It can be difficult to forgive and move on, particularly if you have been badly hurt. Blame is a natural response to the hurt that someone else has caused you. However no one can 'make you' feel anything, unless you allow it. When we refuse to forgive and instead hold on to suffering, hurt and resentment, rather than punishing the other person, what we are doing is punishing ourselves.

We are the ones who hold on to the pain. It is like dragging a ball and chain around with us. We become bitter and untrusting. If we had the wisdom to understand that whoever harmed us was in deep pain themselves, no matter how badly they behaved, then we would have compassion instead of blame. Then we set ourselves free.

As the old adage goes, 'bless your enemy and you rob him of his ammunition'.

Now returning your focus back to your chest, heart and breathing, what do you think you can change that will bring this part of your body back to health? Are there changes to your posture and/or your thinking patterns that you want to make?

Note down any thoughts you have before moving on to the next meditation.

♥ Meditation #5: Loving With All Your Heart

Here is a meditation for you to do when you have a few quiet minutes that will help you to heal your heart and heal any imbalances within your chest. When you are ready and in a relaxed state, ask yourselves these questions. Take time to fully absorb each of the questions, one at a time, and allow the answers to emerge unconsciously

Do you operate from an open heart and express yourself openly and lovingly and fully? Are you living life to the full and being the person you were born to be? Does your heart feel open or closed? Is there any past hurt, pain or resentment still locked within your heart? Are there any hidden feelings from the past that are stopping you from reaching your full potential? Do you have past feelings of inadequacy? Anger? Sorrow? Loneliness? Unfulfilled dreams?

Just feel into the feeling and let your answers rise. Tune into your heart centre and ask it what it's really feeling. What is it that you are hiding from yourself and the world? Let any pain or emotion come to the surface. It wants acknowledgement from you. It wants to heal.

These feelings are from your past, even though you may still be feeling them in the present. The past no longer lives in the present unless you allow it to. It is time to now fully live with an open heart, it is time to let it go, it is time to live in the present again and to create the future you deserve to have, which is free from past hurts and past pain.

Imagine all of those past or present feelings dissolving. It is that simple. All you need to do is to give it permission to let go. This requires you to fully forgive yourself and everyone else for whatever reason their own pain led them to hurt you. Notice any resistance at this point. Is there a part of you not wanting to let it go? Why is this? Be gentle and honest with yourself. What would it mean if you were able to fully forgive and to let go?

Once you are ready to fully let go of your past pain and hurt, take a big deep breath into your tummy and with the out breath, let it go. Feel your abdomen soften and your heart melting as all past blocks and tension disappear. Take your time breathing and letting go as you exhale. Feel your breathing deepen as you let go of your past, opening your heart further. You may feel tears of release as you breathe and let go. Feel all tension melting into the ground as you let it all go.

It is no longer a part of who you are. Open up your heart chakra and imagine there is a big ball of green or pink loving light there. If you find it difficult to feel love, think of someone, something or a pet that you love or that makes you smile. Feel this love growing bigger and bigger within your chest. As you breathe in, you breathe in love and as you breathe out you breathe out love. Allow this feeling to expand to your entire body. When you feel your body full of love, send it outwards to all the people in your past who have hurt you. You forgive them now so you can release yourself and others.

You forgive to be free.

You are now pure, free, loving and confident. Anything is now possible for you. Take a deep breath in, then open your eyes. Notice how expansive and open your chest feels.

Write a positive affirmation or statement that is full of love and forgiveness to help your heart to stay open and repeat this affirmation with your full heart every day or as often as you can remember.

My affirmation to reprogram the language of my chest and heart is:...

....

KEY LESSONS FROM CHAPTER ELEVEN

- **Your heart is a great healer, letting got of the past hurts and resentments you hold in your heart and learning to be open-hearted in the present moment, is vital to your future health, happiness and success**

CHAPTER TWELVE

Your Doing Centre

In this chapter we going to move on from the being centre to the doing centre. As you set your intention for this section of Your MindBody Journey, take a moment to consider this question: "Do you spend more time doing or being?"

How do you balance your activities (your doing time) with your being time, the time when you are still, receptive and relaxed? Most of us are addicted to 'doing' too much, filling our lives with more and more things to entertain ourselves. We get so caught up in the busy-ness of being 'out there' we forget what's going on 'in here'!

When we are too busy to be still and be with the self, we get an inner yearning, an inner discontentment, a feeling of being unfulfilled. When we feel un-ful-filled---we experience ourselves as being empty, as not being filled up enough. To address this emptiness, we go searching for more things to fill up our time, to fill up lives, our minds, our bodies, our diaries until we have enough things to make us feel ful-filled again.

Ironically, this process of filling our lives to make us feel emotionally fulfilled tends to make us feel more unfulfilled. What we are searching for is ourselves, our 'true self'. We miss our soul and the deeper part of who we truly are. Until we understand what's really going on inside of us we will keep searching for the answers outside of us.

For example, we are often attracted to partners because we admire the part of them that is hidden within ourselves, and hasn't been fully expressed. Sometimes we clash with the people we love because of the parts of their character we dislike reminds us of our shadow side, which is the parts of us we don't like about ourselves and try to hide from others, and from ourselves.

The road to fulfilment is always the road to knowing the self. Most of us don't like being still and being with ourselves, because we don't like ourselves. And if we don't fully love and accept ourselves for who we truly are, then we will find that no one else will.

To fully heal and lead a happy fulfilled life, as hard as it is, we need to be still. When we ignore issues or bury our issues, they will always be brought to our attention in some other form, and most of the time, not in pleasant ways, because then we are forced to listen. If we push sickness away or ignore it, we're actually instructing our body not to heal itself. We send messages to our white blood cells that there is nothing wrong, so there is no need to fight the illness, making us more ill. So avoidance is detrimental in more ways than one.

If we have a belief system that we can only love ourselves or be loved once we are perfect, then we will never find love. When we fully love who we are and accept ourselves in all our imperfections, only then can we give unconditional love to others. It is then that we will be truly at peace.

Your shoulders, arms and hands

Your shoulders, arms and hands make up your 'doing' centre and are the channel through which you express what you do in your life through your actions.

Your shoulders are where the active energy from your chest is expressed out into the world via your arms. They are the channel for expressing your true nature. The shoulders get tense and rigid when you aren't expressing your real needs, when you are doing something you would rather not do or doing things because you feel you 'should do'. Your shoulders are the part of your body that carries all your burdens, your troubles and other people's troubles too.

If your shoulders feel tight, then perhaps you are taking on more responsibility than you can handle? The shoulders are used as a protection against getting hurt. Hunching up in anticipation and unconsciously holding your shoulders by your ears is a classic sign of wanting to disappear into your shell. If you do this regularly, then your muscles will be held in a state of constant static contraction. As a result, your energy cannot flow freely and the expression from your heart will be blocked. An extreme version of this leads to conditions like frozen shoulder, which is linked to an inability to give or receive freely.

The Tale Of The Guilty Squash Player

Ben is an accomplished squash player who came to me for a sports remedial massage treatment, to help him with a torn rotator cuff in his right shoulder. Because I am always tuned in to the MindBody connection, I instinctively asked Ben why he thought he had this injury, as I worked on his shoulder.

He looked at me blankly and gave me a very rational, matter-of-fact answer, 'because I tore it playing squash'. So I tried another tack, I asked him what shoulders represented to him. He immediately replied, 'burdens'. I asked him if he felt at all burdened. He went silent, then eventually said, 'I suppose I feel like I'm shouldering the burden of a secret I was told a long time ago'. I encouraged him to go on. He said that he hadn't told anyone about this and felt so burdened with the responsibility of the knowledge of it.

Ben went on to tell me that when his father was on his death bed, he asked Ben to promise to look after his step brother who was then in his late teens. He promised he would, however Ben never really got on with his stepbrother and found it hard to fulfil this promise once his father passed away. I noted to myself that this 'masculine' burden had shown up in the right side of Ben's body, as is often the case.

Since then he felt ashamed and guilty. I asked him if he ever takes this feeling of shame and guilt into his squash tournaments. He said, 'All the time and it affects me so much. There isn't a day that passes when I don't think about it as I feel like I've let my father down'. After the treatment I suggested that he made peace with this burden, to either forgive himself for not fulfilling his promise, or to fulfil the promise.

A few months later, Ben came to see me again and told me that he had contacted his stepbrother and ended up telling him everything, about the promise, about his guilt around not keeping the promise and that he was sorry. His stepbrother was so touched by his honesty that they are now in regular contact. Ben said he felt so different now, so free and untroubled.

He was also pleased that his shoulder was so much better, his squash game was back to its usual standard and he had won his last three tournaments!

Exercise #14:
What Do Your Shoulders Say About You?

Check the posture of your shoulders now. It helps to stand up to do this. Feel how your shoulders connect from your chest to your head. Are they tight? Loose? Rigid? Are they different on the left side to your right side? Are your shoulders arched back or forward at the shoulder joint? What attitude do you think you often adopt to go with your shoulder posture?

Now here is a little game to help you sense how your shoulders act out your emotions. This requires a bit of acting, but don't worry if you don't put in an Oscar-winning performance, in fact this exercise works best if you really overact! Remember, the more you put in the exercise, the more you'll get out of it.

First, act out what your shoulders would do if you were the happiest person in the world. Really express happiness with your shoulders. You can use your whole body to do this, but make sure your shoulders have the lead role.

Now do the same with fear. What do scared shoulders act like? Now try angry shoulders, how would the shoulders of a person filled with anger behave? What about sad shoulders? Make sure you play the part long enough to really feel the sadness in your shoulders.

Now try and act as if your shoulders are disgusted. See if you can act out the most disgusted shoulders in the world. Then move to surprised shoulders, imagine your shoulders belong to a person who is constantly surprised, what does that look and feel like.

Finally, it's time to reprise your happy shoulders, so do your happy shoulders again so you finish this part of the exercise in a good place.

Now stop and tune into your body and consider this question: out of all of these shoulder positions you acted out, which one is most like your natural posture? The posture of your shoulders will help you to get a sense of your character and your emotional history, because this will show up in the habitual position of your shoulders.

Your Shoulders

Here are some more examples of body language that's associated with the shoulders:

Rounded Shoulders: is the weight of the world on your shoulders? Do you tend to take on more responsibilities than you can handle?

Hunched Shoulders: are you protecting yourself? Do you fear being hurt? Are you a shallow breather?

Raised Shoulders: are you wanting to disappear? Are you a tortoise wanting to retreat into your shell? Where did you experience fear in the past? Your original fear may have gone, but you may tend to project the old fear on to new objects.

Square Shoulders: are you concerned with the way you appear in the world? Do you want to appear bigger or more powerful than you actually feel?

Slight Shoulders: are you afraid to express yourself? Do you have an underdeveloped ego?

Frozen Shoulder: are you able to give and receive freely in equal measures? Are you doing what you love in life? Are you hugging the right person?

Write down what you think your shoulders say about you. Then ask yourself what you can change to bring your shoulders into balance, by changing your posture and/or thinking patterns?

Write a positive affirmation or statement and read it every day or as often as you can remember. Remember to 'feel' the words instead of just saying the words. This will help to create a new, positive, resourceful neural pathway.

My affirmation to reprogram the language of my shoulders is:..

....

Your Arms And Hands

You arms and hands represent the way you give and receive, they are your channels for expression. The health of your arms, elbows and hands are dependent on the ability to express feelings in giving and receiving into action.

There is a natural law of giving (masculine energy) and receiving (feminine energy). This doesn't mean only men give and only women receive, rather that we all have masculine giving energy and feminine receiving energy within us.

In Eastern tradition this energy has been known for millennia as Yin (feminine) and Yang (masculine). Where Yin and Yang are in perfect balance then your body and mind will feel balanced and harmonious.

The universe operates in cycles of inhalations (feminine, yin, receiving) and exhalations (masculine, yang, giving). When you only give or only receive, then you become out of rhythm with your natural flow and the flow of life. We see the natural law of giving and receiving (Yin and Yang, feminine and masculine) operating everywhere in the natural world. Baby animals and birds receive food from their parents to survive, then later in return they give to their young to keep them alive. In the summer we see the rain giving to the soil and the soil receiving it to nourish the new crops. The male sperm gives to the female egg, the egg in return opens to receive the sperm.

In nature, the oak tree doesn't get angry when a squirrel takes its acorn. The leaf doesn't fear dropping in the Autumn or prevent the soil from receiving nourishment from the fallen leaf. The natural world knows of the law of unconditional giving and receiving, because if it didn't give, then it wouldn't receive, and then there would be no life. The natural world works in perfect harmony and each element works together to support life for the whole.

We humans, on the other hand, don't often work within the same law. We fear we won't be provided for, so we become greedy and hoard things. We fear that if we give, we will be without. We fear that if we receive we will be seen as selfish.

Do you give and receive with the natural flow of the universe, or do you force and take and work against the rhythms of nature? Do you operate within the natural law of balance, which is to give and receive with no hidden agendas, giving and receiving unconditionally from your heart, with no fears attached? When we are in fear, then our giving becomes forcing and our receiving becomes taking. There is a profound difference between 'taking' and 'receiving', between 'forcing' and 'giving'. Receiving and giving are working with a natural flow. Forcing and taking are resisting and conflicting energies, which go against a natural flow.

When I was learning about the natural laws of giving and receiving, I had an experience that tested the theory. I was on a camping holiday and had just been on a big supermarket shop for all the food I needed for a week. I put the cold food in the shared camp kitchen fridge and a little voice inside me said, 'Are you sure it'll be safe in there?' I pushed the thought aside and worked on my belief that everyone was trustworthy.

The next morning I went to the fridge to get my breakfast and in horror I noticed that all my food had gone! Every bit of it had been stolen! I stood there for ages with my mouth gaping open not sure of how to react! I was monitoring my thoughts, feelings and reactions, and in the end I took a couple of deep breaths and decided to send my blessings to whoever took my food, deciding that they obviously needed it more than me.

As I walked out of the camp kitchen, there on the ground in front of me was a $50 note, the exact amount of money I spent on the food the previous day! I looked around me to see if it belonged to anyone, but there was no one in sight. This to me was evidence that when I graciously gave with no resistance, then I would naturally receive.

Do you operate within the natural laws of giving and receiving in equal amounts? Or are you more of a giver? If so why? Are you more of a receiver? If so why? When you give and receive, do you do it from your heart or are there conditions? Be honest with yourself as these are important questions to ponder on. Your answers could signal a breakthrough in the way you approach life.

MindBody Arm Language

Here are some MindBody symptoms related to your arms and hands. Do any relate to you? If so write them down.

Weak Underdeveloped Arms: are you holding on to energy and expression in your chest, belly or shoulders? Are you able to reach out and take hold of life?

Big Arm Muscles: do you relate to others in an insensitive way, using force to hold onto things?

Fat Arms: do you feel a deadness or sluggishness in your actions, an apathy and your heart really isn't in it?

Thin Tight Arms: do you grasp or clutch onto things? Do you find you are able to reach out to people but you have difficulty in holding on to anything?

Right Arm: this is your masculine, giving side. If there are issues or problems in your right arm or hand this may indicate problems, resistance or resentment in how you give in life.

Left Arm: this is your feminine, receiving side. If there are issues in your left arm or hand, this may indicate problems, resistance or resentment in how you receive in life.

Elbow Problems: do you have disjointed energy? Are you saying one thing and doing another?

Getting To Know Your Hands

Your hands are powerful transmitters of your emotional state. If you get excited notice how they tingle. Healers will tell you that their hands get hot or tingly when they give healing. This is their electromagnetic energy. We all have it, but we are not perhaps aware of it. If a child gets hurt, the mother or father intuitively wants to rub and hold the injured area, which transmits these powerful healing energies.

You often show your energy in motion (e-motion) in your body language. If you are upset or fearful, you withdraw your arms. When you are happy and positive you open your arms. These are limbic responses programmed within you from your ancient ancestors. Arms and hands are the channel for your expressions of giving and receiving. They express how you are 'being' when you are 'doing' the act of giving or receiving, they are the emotions behind the action.

Cold Hands: do you have a difficulty in reaching out to people and accepting help?

Clammy Hands: do you feel powerless in relationships or to people and things?

Here are some questions to ask yourself.

Are you doing what you want in life or is that expression blocked? Are you expressing your feelings into action?

Are you fully able to give and receive. Why do you do what you do in life? What is the intention behind what you do?

What posture or muscle issues have you adopted in your arms and hands as a result of your attitude? Attitudes around giving and receiving and your ability to express yourself? Are you 'doing' what you want in life? Do you equally give and receive with no agenda? Are you too much of a giver, or too much of a receiver? Do you give to yourself and receive for yourself unconditionally? Or do you block this natural flow?

What have you discovered about your arms and hands? What do you think this represents? What do your think you can change?

Talking To Your Unconscious Mind

There is a holistic therapy called Kinesiology that was developed by Dr George Goodheart, combining modern Western techniques and knowledge drawn from Eastern health systems. Kinesiology is a muscle testing technique to monitor the flow of energy throughout the body. Through this system a kinesiologist practitioner can identify the factors which may be disrupting the natural flow of energy which are essential for good health. By testing the muscle with 'yes' or 'no' responses, the body can tell us the answers to virtually anything!

The body stores memory and this is a really good method of tapping into our unconscious to retrieve that memory. I have used kinesiology to find out what vitamins my body needs, what house was best suited for me to live in, to even finding out the actual time of my birth, which was later confirmed by my mother to be true. The body never lies.

If you have a partner handy, you can ask your body some questions, as long as they are framed in a way that can be answered 'yes' or 'no'.

Exercise #15:
How To Access Your Inner Truth

The person who wants the answers (Person A) stands with their feet hip width apart with their right arm outstretched to their side parallel to the floor, holding the arm firm but not tight. The other person (Person B) stands behind them and places their left hand on Person A's right shoulder, and their other hand at the end of Person A's out-stretched arm, over their wrist.

First we need to establish a 'yes' and 'no' system which tells us if the body has power (our life force) or has lost its power. Person B tests the strength of Person A's out-stretched arm by gently pressing it down, Person A slightly resists the pressure.

Now you have established what feels 'strong'.

Person A then says their name out loud, 'My name is _____'. Person B tests the arm strength by again gently pushing the arm down. The arm should test strong. Now person A says a different name, 'My name is_____' (using a false name like 'Ermentrude' or 'Tarquin'). Person B should notice that the strength or power in person A's arm goes weak, by again gently pressing their arm down. The arm will feel like it has lost power, lost its life force. This is how our body responds when we are thinking, feeling and saying things that are 'true' and 'false'.

Do you remember our exercise at the beginning of the book when your body felt weak when you had negative thoughts and the body felt strong when you had positive thoughts? Kinesiology works on the same principle.

Now you can ask the body anything you want, making sure to ask questions that require yes or no answers. For example if Person A asks, 'Is chocolate good for me?' and the arm goes weak then you can be sure it is a 'no' answer. If you ask 'What is causing my headaches?' you won't get your answer. Here you will need to go through questions of elimination, like, 'Is lack of sleep the cause of my headaches?' Then you will get your 'yes' or 'no' response.

If you don't have a partner at hand, you can do this exercise by yourself by 'tuning' in to your body energy. You can 'feel' your body go weak if it is a 'no' answer and you can 'feel' your body go strong on a 'yes' answer. You might find your body leans forward slightly to 'yes' answers or leans back to 'no' answers. Just ask the question and wait to see what your body does to give you a yes/no response.

Once you tune into these feelings regularly (this is your intuition and your gut feelings) then you will become masterful at making decisions your 'inner self' knows are right for you.

The Tale Of The Surprisingly Angry Lady

A client came to see me regarding a pain in her arm. It wasn't getting better even after a few treatments, so I asked her what emotion her arm was wanting to release? And because it was her right arm I asked her what action her arm was being repressed from doing. She immediately said, 'hitting!'

She was a very patient and kind lady and not the sort of person that normally went around hitting things. Her emotions however were at boiling point with a person in her life and she did indeed want to hit them. Because she was repeatedly suppressing an action from a rising emotion, the energy stayed within her body and created a muscle block. She tried lots of displacement activities like going for long walks, shaking her arms about and even using her scatter cushions as an impromptu punch bag, but it wasn't until she found a way to deal with the person she wanted to hit, that the pain went away.

I'm not saying we must always act upon our emotions, but it is healthy to acknowledge or release the emotions in a way that is appropriate for us, and ideally to find a way to address the underlying issue.

Exercise #16:
Open Up Your Arms

Here are some physical exercises for your shoulders, arms and hands. They will help to loosen all of your muscles, release any energy blocks and help let go of the mind set attached to these blocks. However, if you have any injuries in your arms or shoulders then listen to your body to assess your safe limits, but also be aware of the fear behind your limitations which might be dictating to you. Learn to become discerning to the voices in your head. Do they come from a place of love or do they come from a place of fear? It is important that you keep your body relaxed and don't brace yourself throughout the exercises.

Read through the instructions below first.

Stand tall in Mountain Pose with your legs slightly apart and your arms by your side. Start to rotate your shoulders up, round and back a few times and then up, round and forward. How do they feel? Are they loose, tight or inflexible? Now take a deep breath in and raise your shoulders up to your ears, shrugging your shoulders and with a loud out breath, let your shoulders drop down letting go of any stress, burdens and fears. Do this as many times as you need to, or until your mind is clear.

Next, clasp your hands behind your back and keeping your arms and upper body straight, raise your clasped hands upwards. This helps to open up your heart and stretches the pectoral muscle in your chest. Hold for as long as you need to get benefit from the stretch.

Now start to swing your right arm backwards and forwards, allowing the energy in your arm to flow. When you're ready, swing your arm round and round in big circles, brushing past your ear with enough speed for it to start to gain its own momentum. Then stop and repeat this big, circling motion in the opposite direction. Do this for as long as you feel you need to. Then take a deep breath in and with the exhale, flick your arm as if flicking off an unwanted insect.

Flick the whole arm using a loud, fast exhale to release any old unwanted, stuck energy related to giving. Keep going until your whole shoulder joint feels loose and relaxed.

Come to a stop with both arms to your sides and notice how different your right arm feels to your left. Describe this feeling in words. You may also notice your right arm is now longer than the other! This is the result of freeing all the tendons and ligaments around your joints. Now do the same with your left arm. This time letting go of any old, stuck issues related to receiving. After you have completed the exercise with both arms, notice how both arms feel.

Now you have got to know your doing centre a little better, what do your shoulders, arms and hands say about you? Are you able to express yourself easily through your actions by giving and receiving freely and doing what you love?

During the exercises, was there any discomfort, resistance or inflexibility in your shoulders or arms? What was the feeling behind the discomfort? What do you think this represents for you? Write down your answers.

What can you change, by altering your posture and/or thinking patterns, to bring your mind and body back into a healthy balance?

♥ Meditation #6:
Letting Yourself Go With The Flow

Here is a meditation which will help you to clear any tension, tightness or emotional blocks held within your doing centre. Read through it first, or get someone to read it to you. Allow at least 20 minutes of quiet time.

Get into a comfortable position, preferably lying down with your arms out from your sides. Take some deep breaths and wait for your mind to settle by focusing on your breath. When you are relaxed and ready bring your attention to your shoulders and your arms and tune into any tension, tightness or energy blocks that are there.

Listen to that tightness and what it might be saying. Allow that part of the body to speak to you. If your shoulders had a voice, what would they say to you right now? Listen to the first answers that come up. Stay quiet and still and let your body speak to you.

Now bring your awareness to your right arm, your giving self, and listen. What does this arm want to say to you? What hidden messages are stored there regarding your ability to give? Take your time to really listen.

Now bring your awareness to your left arm, your receiving self, and listen. What does your left arm want to say to you? What hidden messages are stored in your left arm regarding your ability to receive? Again take your time.

So now image your energy flowing easily and freely from your chest. Breathe in from your chest, and send it up to your shoulders then send it down your right arm with the out breath and then out through your hand. Breathe in and out in a continuous flow through your shoulders and down your right arm. Giving is easy and rewarding, it feels good to give of yourself and share your gifts with the world. It feels great when you are able to assert your need to give all you want to give.

Imagine that your right arm is now free and able to express itself fully.

Now imagine energy flowing easily and freely from your left hand, starting from the tips of your fingers with the in breath, and up your left arm to your shoulders on the out breath, down into your heart in a continuous flow. You are worthy of receiving all you deserve and all you wish for. It is your birthright that you are able to give and receive in a constant, continuous flow. Feel the energy flowing freely in through your left arm to your heart. It feels wonderful to receive the abundance of the universe and bring it inside of you.

Imagine that your left arm is now free and fully able to receive.

With your next in breath, imagine the energy flowing from your heart and out through both your arms out into the your life with no fear. There are no restrictions, you are safe to give to the world all your love, gifts and talents. Breathe into your heart filling it up with all your love, gifts and talents, now breathing that abundance of yourself out into the world.

Now imagine this energy coming back to you tenfold. Everything you have ever wanted is coming to you through your open arms. Open yourself up to receive. Receiving all your heart's desires. Feel your chest expand and your body filling up, tingling with this energy. Now combine the two.

With every in breath you receive and with every out breath you give. See this energy in a circular rhythmic flow, coming out from you and back to you. It is energy which is real and you can feel it flowing through you now. Make this feeling and this energy as big as you can. Make it bigger than you, bigger than the room, bigger than the street and the town you're in, bigger than your country and the world, make it bigger than the solar system and as big as the whole universe. Your giving and receiving energy is an infinite source of power and abundance, it's only you that blocks it. Know this power is always there to serve you.

With this new energy built up inside you, you can now take it into your life with a sense of freedom and abundance as all your heart's desires are now coming to you effortlessly. When you are ready, bring your awareness back into the room and notice how your doing centre feels.

Now write your positive affirmation or statement and read this affirmation every day or as often as you can remember.

My affirmation to reprogram the language of my arms and hands is:...

....

KEY LESSONS FROM CHAPTER TWELVE

- **Your doing centre is your channel for giving and receiving, keep this channel open if you want to live an abundant and expressive life**

CHAPTER THIRTEEN

Your Control Centre

This is the final chapter in Part Two of Your MindBody Journey. In this section we will be taking a closer look at your 'control centre', which comprises your neck, face and head and brain. Take a moment to set your intention for this part of the journey and once you are ready, we'll start by discussing how you can learn to control the muscles in every part of your body.

Do you have any muscle aches and pains? Notice how you hold your muscles when you are doing an everyday activity, like cleaning your teeth, filling up the kettle, driving your car or even sitting watching TV. Are your muscles tense or relaxed? Are you using muscles you don't need to, like your jaw, your shoulders or your buttocks for doing simple tasks?

It is amazing how many people unconsciously hold onto muscles they don't need to, causing the muscle to statically contract. Your neurological pathways have learnt this behaviour. This leads to all sorts of problems.

I spent years as a therapist doing remedial body work. Most of the people who came to see me because of a strained muscle, were not the sports players, or labourers, but people who lived fairly sedentary lifestyles. Sore necks, shoulders or bad backs are often caused by holding our body in one position for a long time, constantly contracting a muscle or muscle group. Most of the time my clients were not aware they were doing this, as it is an unconscious learnt behaviour. With these people, I usually work with their mind before their body, as there is no point fixing an issue in the body, only for it to come back again. And If we keep thinking the same thoughts in our minds, then we keep creating the same problems in our bodies.

If you think you are one of these people, internally scan your muscles now and check if any are tight and not relaxed. If there is any tightness, then you need to mentally keep reminding yourself, 'is my arm/ shoulder/ jaw relaxed?'. If it isn't then learn to relax it when prompted. The best way to do this is tighten your muscle or your whole body first, then with the out breath, let your muscles relax.

The more you do this, the more your body will learn how to be relaxed. It is amazing how the body forgets to relax if you don't remind it! Leave messages or a symbol around your house or office, or wherever you spend most of your time and every time you see the word 'relax' or the symbol you have chosen, your body will be prompted to relax. If you practice this every-day, religiously, it wont be long before your neural pathway has been rewired and your old muscle programming has been replaced by your new muscle programming. Many studies have shown it takes about 21 days to create a new pathway, at which point, you no longer need to consciously remind yourself because your new way of holding your body, has now become an unconscious habit.

You can apply this to any old habit you have in your life that no longer works for you. You may have a habit of craving food, cigarettes or other body addictions and because you repeat the habit over and over, it forms a brain pathway. However your brain is always changing and you can forge a new pathway and create new habits.   The brain is very much like exercising a muscle, the more you move a muscle the bigger it gets and if you don't use a muscle it fades away.

Therefore when you change your mind and your way of thinking, connections that relate to your old way dissolve and connections that correspond to your new way of thinking begin to grow. The results are dependent on how committed you are and how much you want to change your habits.

Your Neck

Your neck is the major channel where your brain communic-ates with the rest of your body, it continually mediates between your thoughts and your feelings, your head and your heart.

Do you have problems making decisions? Do you hear a 'yes' from your heart then your rational brain kicks in telling you all the reasons to say 'no'? When your thoughts and feelings are not in alignment it results in separation. Conflict between your head and heart results in a MindBody split. This is where the expression a 'pain in the neck' comes from.

When you feel emotions (energy in motion), the energy flows up from your belly and chest, then is expressed through your arms (action) and/or enters your neck, where your feelings are translated into thoughts and words. If, however this energy is not expressed, then it can get stuck in your neck. Therefore, sore or tight neck muscles are often found in people who like to be in control. Fear is always behind control issues. The function of your neck muscles is to enable your head to turn from side to side, so if you have a tight or restricted mobility in your neck, what does this tell you about the way you see the world? Are you able to see all sides and from all angles of life? Or do you fear seeing what's on the other side?

Your neck houses your throat chakra. If your throat chakra is blocked you are probably holding back in some way and fearful of expressing yourself openly and honestly. Physically this will affect your throat, your breathing and your thyroid gland. As children most of us were taught that there are 'good' emotions and 'bad' emotions, and that it is best not to express bad emotions. We have been conditioned into displaying only 'appropriate' emotions to fit in with society's expectations. We often get angry inside but don't allow ourselves an outlet for this anger. When emotions are avoided, they are pushed out of sight into our 'shadow' side but they don't disappear. They follow us around, lurking in our shadow, until that side of us is expressed in some potentially unhealthy way. This is why all sides of our humanity need a healthy outlet of expression.

Think back to when you were a child and remember how you were in your true spirit before you learnt not to be. Were you able to openly express what you were feeling or were you told to suppress certain feelings? Was there a specific event or a time that you can remember when you were ashamed, sad, stopped or told off for fully expressing yourself emotionally? What impact has that had on the rest of your life? Have you blocked certain emotional expression? If so you may suffer from coughs, tonsillitis, tight jaws or grinding teeth.

The throat Chakra is the first 'spiritual' chakra. It marks the beginning of your deeper understanding of yourself. Who are you? What do you know about your real self? What are your strengths and your weaknesses? Are you satisfied with who you are? Do you openly express yourself or do you behave how you believe others want you to be?

What does your neck and throat say about you? Write down your answers.

Your Face

You are capable of over ten thousand different facial expressions! Your face is a map of all the experiences you've ever had. You can often see in an elderly person's face, the story of the type of life they have led, by their permanently fixed expression. If they have a lot of laughter lines, they have experienced a lot of joy. If their brow is furrowed, they have frowned a lot and had a life marked by worry. If their mouth turns upwards, they have generally put on a happy face. If their mouth turns down, they have probably experienced a lot of misery. If you're worried about how you'll look when you are old, try to stop worrying because it will give you wrinkles and smile instead, it's cheaper than a facelift!

So what consistent thoughts have you held to create the permanent expressions of your face? Are you facing up to facts? Are you saving face? What is your face saying to the people you meet? We make our first impression with our face. What is your usual expression? A bright smiling face? A sad and grumpy face? What message are you giving others? This is your mask that you put on each day and share with the world. Is your mask true or false? If you have tension in your jaw and face, it is usually a sign that you are acting out a false story instead of showing your true feelings. Are you grinding and mulling and not expressing what you really think?

What does your face say about you?
Write down your answers.

Your Forehead

Your forehead is where your third eye chakra is located, which is situated in the space between your eyebrows. It is where you see clearly beyond your physical sight. It is your heightened sense of self-awareness, your sixth sense.

Everyone has this sixth sense, how many times have you heard yourself say something like 'I knew that was going to happen'? This is often our sixth sense in action, we all have it, it's just most of us haven't been taught to use this psychic ability so it's weak or non-existent, just like a muscle that hasn't been exercised for years.

When you are weighed down with fear you cannot access more expansive insights. Whether you believe it or not, you are connected to all things and not separate and alone, you are part of a mass consciousness. But it is your ego that holds on to separateness. All your answers are within you, within your instincts and intuition, it's just a case of learning to trust and follow them.

Is there a difference between instinct and intuition? I believe that instinct is our ancient programmed survival mechanism. It is the part of us that learnt to keep us safe from danger in our ancestral past. I personally believe instincts belong to the human consciousness, whereas intuition belongs to our soul consciousness. Intuition is our deeper knowing, a 'feeling' an inner knowing and wisdom.

It comes from your heart and from a place of trust, when fear isn't nagging you. Intuition is that deep-seated inner feeling that just 'knows' something is right. When we are not in tune with our intuition and inner knowing, we usually let our brain run the show, and because we live only five percent of the time from our conscious mind, it's no wonder we make the wrong choices! Not being connected to our intuition, can be like being enveloped by thick fog. How would it feel if you were continually surrounded by real fog, day in day out, year after year? Would you accept that this is all there is? Would you believe, there was no view, no vision beyond the fog? No clear picture of what lies ahead?

This is how most of us live our everyday lives, in the fog! Yet if we trusted our inner 'knowing', the inner wisdom of our internal compass, we would know that there is something beyond the fog. Have you ever had this feeling before? If so, did you act upon it? And when you did, did everything work out just perfectly?

Exercise #17:
How To Reprogram Your Mind

The next exercise, inspired by Thomas Hanna's book 'Somatics', will lessen sore or tight neck muscles. It will help to retrain your neck and head muscles to respond independently allowing your energy to flow freely. This helps to reprogram the sensory motor section of your brain, developing your ability to see all sides, broadening your view and breaking patterns of limited thinking. It is the outer change in muscle function that makes possible inner changes to brain function, by breaking habitual patterns.

It's best to do this exercise standing up and make sure you are gentle with your neck only stretching it as far as is comfortable and right for you.

Start by turning your head to one side as far as it will comfortably go and note how far your head turns (by spotting where your nose is in relation to your shoulder). Bring your head back to facing forward. Now turn your head the same side and this time move your eyes to look as far as you can over your shoulder. Notice how much further you went. Now swap sides.

Now turn your head to the side again, but this time make your eyes look in the opposite direction. How easy was this to do? Also notice how your neck muscles responded. Now turn your head to the other side and look in the opposite direction. Your neck muscles are used to operating simultaneously with your eyes. This exercise will help them to learn to work independently from the eyes, breaking the pattern of tightness in your neck and shoulders.

Lift your face up to the ceiling, then back down towards your chest. Repeat five times. Now lift your face up to the ceiling and at the same time you look down to the floor. Now bring your chin down towards your chest and look up. Repeat five times. How easy do you find this? The more difficult you find these movements, then the more likely it is that your existing patterning and programming is fixed and rigid.

Now let's try one last exercise, this is my favourite. Rotate you head slowly and as you do, notice how your eyes tend to follow the circle you are drawing with your nose. Now try again and as you do, keep moving your eyes to look in the opposite direction to where the movement is heading. So when your nose heads right, your eyes look left. When your nose points up, you look down, and so on.

Apart from looking really weird as you do this (I wouldn't do this in a public place if you don't want to be stared at!) it's a really good exercise to help you to break free from patterning. Breaking your patterning is vital to the transformation process. Breaking your patterns sometimes requires you to step out of your comfort zone, but by breaking your habitual patterns, it will be easier to rewire your programming.

There are different ways you can do this. Start with a small change, like driving or walking a different way to work. Wear different coloured clothing to what you would normally wear, or try different food, read a different type of book or newspaper, listen to a different radio station or watch a TV show you don't normally watch. Once doing different things becomes easy for you, why not consider taking an even bigger step out of your comfort zone, like doing a sponsored sky dive or public speaking or handing in your notice?

What are you not doing that you'd really love to try? Is it time to break the pattern and step outside your comfort zone to do something different? Don't keep it to yourself, make a commitment to do something new and different and tell a friend when you're going to do it and then ask them to support you by making sure you follow it through.

The Crown Chakra

Situated at the top of your head is your crown chakra. This is where your energy is very pure and enlightened. It is your place of awakening. When you fully awaken, you operate primarily from your soul as opposed to from your ego and from your suffering. It is fully opened when all your MindBody tensions have been dissolved. From self consciousness comes cosmic consciousness. In life you will go through some hefty life experiences (I call them initiations) to lighten your load towards true inner peace and happiness. You'll go through many stages of self consciousness, each processed through the chakras, from your base to your crown chakra.

You have been working through and opening up each chakra on Your MindBody Journey, as you have released your limiting thoughts relating to each body centre and chakra and learnt to express your true self, instead of operating through the persona you have built up for protection.

Your Head And Brain

Your head sits on top of your spine and it weighs approximately five pounds. That's the same as five bags of sugar, or 2 litres of milk!!! Your neck muscles do an amazing job of supporting your head so that it sits effortlessly on the top of your spine. However, because most of us develop a poor posture, our head is too far forward and over time this will disrupt this fine balance. Every inch that your head is forward, the weight load on your neck and spine increases by another ten pounds. That's like balancing an extra ten bags of sugar or four and a half litres (eight pints) of milk on top of our heads. No wonder most of us have sore necks and shoulders.

Your head contains your two brains, by which I mean your right and left cerebral hemispheres. These are linked by the corpus callosum, a big bundle of nerves that communicate to each other. The left side of the brain is responsible for the right side of your body (masculine) and the right side of your brain is responsible for the left side (feminine).

Your brain is the control centre of your entire body. It controls thoughts, memory, speech, and movement. It regulates the function of many organs. Neuroscientists at the university in Palma, Italy, scanned the brains of volunteers who were watching other people move various parts of their body. Amazingly the areas of the brain that controlled the movement of these various parts of the body were activated as if they were the ones doing the movements.

This proves that the brain mirrors what we pay attention to. If someone is sad for instance and you were watching them be sad, your brain will actually think you are sad too. The brain is incredibly sensitive to what we are aware of. Even when we just think about a movement, our brain is stimulated as if we are performing that movement.

In some cases this leads to people having phantom pains and symptoms of illness when a loved one is sick. Your brain doesn't know the difference between what's real and what's imaginary. This means we have the power to imagine ourselves healthy and well, even if we're not, the brain believes that we really are!

When the brain is healthy, it works quickly and automatically. However, when problems occur, the results can be devastating. Brain diseases seem to be getting more wide spread, inflammation in the brain, strokes, brain tumours, Alzheimer's etc. If you are suffering from any of them, then here are some questions you might like to ask yourself. Are you wanting to get out of your mind? Are you wanting to escape from the 'normal' reality of your life? Are you wanting to forget who you are? Your past? Are you resisting old age? Do you want to exit from all your human responsibilities?

MindBody Head And Neck Language

Here are some classic head and neck postures. Do any of these relate to you?

Head Forward: usually means you tend to encounter the world with your head first, with your rational self, then later with your feeling self. Do you check out the danger first before your body feels it is safe to follow?

Long Neck: these are often considered graceful. Are you confident and a proud?

Downward Tilted Neck: do you have difficulty in facing up to the demands and needs of everyday living?

Bull's Neck: do you have a tight and aggressive approach to life's demands?

Ear Problems: what is it you don't want to hear and are not facing up to?

Eye Problems: what is it you are avoiding seeing?

Forehead Issues: are you over thinking and not relaxing enough?

Headaches: are usually caused by restricted blood flow from the neck. Are you holding onto anger? Is your mind in alignment with your heart?

Migraines: are you resisting the flow of life?

What do your head and neck say about you? Write down your answers.

Exercise #18:
Tapping Your Way To Happiness

If you can do this next exercise on a regular basis, you will feel an improvement to the quality of your life, particularly the way you handle stress. They use this BodyTalk System™ in schools to help children with trauma and it is used worldwide. It will help you to repair and rewire the brain, correcting any 'blown fuses' and reconnecting both hemispheres of your brain. It is also beneficial if you suffer from headaches, neck pain, depression, bad circulation, arthritis and hormone imbalances.

In this exercise you use the energy in your hands to connect both hemispheres of your brain. Rub your hands together first and place your hands either side of your head, above your ears and feel the energy flowing between your hands. Now place your left hand on the back of your head and tap the top of your head using your right hand with your fingers wide open. Do this for a few breaths. Then with your right hand, tap your sternum (breast bone). Now move your left hand from the back of your head, to the top of your head and with your other hand tap your forehead. Do this for a few breaths then again tap your sternum. Now move your left hand down to your forehead and with your right hand tap the back of your head, and once again, tap your sternum. Now bring both your hands to the sides of your head, let go of one hand and tap one side of your head and then your sternum. Swap hands and tap the other side of your head and then your sternum.

Finish the exercise with both hands cupping the sides of your head and feel the energy between your hands creating a connection between both brain hemispheres. Now relax and notice how you feel.

Emotional Freedom Technique

There is another tapping technique called EFT (emotional freedom technique) which is brilliant to use if you have a particular fear or phobia. This tapping short circuits your meridians to get them flowing again and you will find that the fear or phobia miraculously disappears.

Firstly name your fear. Then note where you feel it in your body. Rate how severe your fear is on a scale of one to ten (ten being the worst fear your can imagine). Now tap at the start points of your meridians on one side, while focusing on your issue. These are the centre of your eyebrow, the side of your eye, under your eye, under your nose, on your chin, on your chest, at the sides of your ribs where your bra strap runs (if you wear one) and at the top of your crown.

Tap the points while talking about and describing your fear. For example, 'even though my chest is tight and I feel anxious and sick in my stomach when I think about speaking in public, I feel safe to feel this, and even though I feel this anxiety, I love and accept myself and my feelings'. Keep tapping and talking about the feelings out loud until you notice the feelings start to subside. Once you have tapped and talked for a few rounds, ask yourself what level of your fear is now on a scale of one to ten? Keep repeating the process until the score is at a level you are happy with.

What did you notice about your control centre in these exercises? Was there any discomfort or resistance? If so, what were the feelings behind this? What does this say about you? Write down your answers. Now ask yourself what you can change altering your posture and/or your thinking patterns to bring your mind and body back into a healthy balance? It is now time to write your affirmation regarding your discoveries of your head and neck.

My affirmation to reprogram the language of my head and neck is: ....

....

♥ Meditation #7: Uniting Your MindBody

This meditation is a standing meditation designed to unite all your centres, reflect on your reprogramming and help you to embody your new way of being. You will need a clear space of around 6 ft in front of you, so clear any tables or chairs away. You can read the instructions as you go, but be sure to pause and close your eyes when you need to, to take full advantage of the meditation. Allow at least 20 minutes.

Firstly stand in your new corrected posture (refer to the biofeedback neuromuscular training on page 92 if you need reminding) and tune into your centre of gravity, your hara. Breathe into your belly. You are feeling strong but very relaxed, comfortable and in balance. If not, adjust your body weight until your leg muscles feel balanced and the weight is in the middle of your feet. You feel grounded and in your power.

Take a couple of deep breaths and relax into the posture. Just take a note of how you feel. Tune into your body as a whole. How is it feeling? Cast your mind back to how you felt at the beginning of this book and remember how your mind and your body was feeling then. How does your mind and body feel today? Does your mind feel different? Does your body feel different? If so, what is different? Note how far you have come on Your MindBody Journey and be aware of your potential to be the person you were born to be.

Now bring your consciousness and your awareness into your MOVING CENTRE. This is your hips, legs and feet. This represents your self-support, your stability, your direction and your path forward. Tune into any tightness, weakness, imbalance, issue or energy block you may have discovered in this area during your journey. What is it saying to you? Acknowledge it and let it know it has been heard. Take as much time as you need to reflect. When you feel you are ready, then it is time to finally let that imbalance go. Take a whole breath in and then with the out breath take one tiny but powerful step forward, and leave that old patterning behind.

It is now behind you.

Now tune into your BEING CENTRE. This is your trunk, your tummy, chest and back. This area represents your feelings, your life force, your will, your power and how you are BEING. Tune into any tightness, weakness, imbalance, issue or energy block you may have discovered in this area during your journey. Feel into it. What is it saying to you? Acknowledge it and let it known it has been heard. Take as much time as you need to reflect. When you feel you are ready, then it is time to let that imbalance go. Take a whole breath in and then with the out breath, take one tiny but powerful step forward, and leave that old patterning behind.

It is now behind you.

Now tune into your DOING centre. This is your arms and shoulders. They represent the doing part of who you are. How you are expressing who you are out there into the world. Are you doing what you want in life or is that expression blocked? Are you expressing your feelings into action? Are you fully able to give and receive? Tune into any tightness, weakness, imbalance, issue or energy block you may have discovered in this area during your journey. Feel into it. What is it saying to you? Acknowledge it and let it know it has been heard. Take as much time as you need to reflect. When you are ready, is time to let that imbalance go. Take a whole breath in and with the out breath take one tiny but powerful step forward, and leave the old patterning behind.

It is now behind you.

Now tune into your CONTROL centre. This is your head and neck. I am now going to ask you some questions and just answer the questions internally. The first response is your truth. If you don't have words or an answer, just listen, really listen and tune into your body and notice if there is any discomfort or lowering of your energy within your body to any of the questions, no matter how subtle. You may notice a twitch in your face, a quickening of your breath, a sinking feeling in your tummy, a tightening of the jaw, a lump in your throat, or just a 'knowing' feeling within you. Trust your inner knowing. Trust your inner voice.

Do you feel out of control? What or who do you feel you need to control? What fear is behind that control? If you didn't have a need to control, how would that make your body feel and how would it make your life different? Are you torn between your head and heart? Do you believe in who you are? Are you following the path of your own truth? Are you in alignment? Do you walk your talk? Are you the person you were born to be? Do you do what you love? Is your self-talk supporting or sabotaging your dreams? What limited beliefs have you created that are stopping you from reaching your potential? Take as much time as you need to reflect.

When you are ready, it is time to let those imbalances go. Take a deep breath in and with the out breath take one tiny but powerful step forward, and leave the old patterning behind. You have now let go of past limitations and old patterns that no longer serve you. Allow your body to now feel what it would feel like with no limitations, no restrictions, just being the person you were born to be. Really feel it within your whole body. Imagine how you would walk, talk, act and feel. Notice your posture adjusting to match this. Know you can be this person once your mind and body is free from past programming. Note how free your mind and body are now.

This final step will be one of focus, attention and intention, stepping mindfully into a possible future which is free from past limitations. WITH YOUR MIND AND BODY now take a deep breath in. With the out breath you now take a step forward into your future potential. A future that is centred, powerful and balanced and full of possibility. Feel it in the whole of your being. Embrace it. BE IT, BECAUSE IT IS YOU.

Tune into how your mind and body is feeling and take this forward into the final part of Your MindBody Journey.

KEY LESSONS FROM CHAPTER THIRTEEN

- **Your head is your control centre, it can hold you back or you can use it to set you free. Be mindful of whether your control centre is helping or hindering you in life**

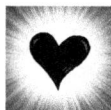

PART THREE: Your Soul

You have now arrived at the final stage of Your MindBody Journey.

Throughout this journey, you've spent much of your time focussing your attention within. In this section of the book you will begin to shift your attention without, as you prepare to consider the bigger picture.

You are part of a greater consciousness, a collective oneness through which you can connect to your ever-present soul. Your life is a constant process of co-creation with the universe, as every thought, word and emotion shapes the life you live.

In this section of the book you will bring Your MindBody Journey to completion, but the best is yet to come. As you prepare to let go of your old programming that no longer works for you and to look forward to a bright, new beginning that does.

CHAPTER FOURTEEN

Your Thoughts And Beliefs

It is said that on average you will have around 50,000 thoughts a day, with as many as 95% of those thoughts being the same thoughts as you had yesterday! If most of those 50,0000 thoughts are negative or repetitive then nothing will change in your life.

Remember the thoughts you think, give you the body you embody, and the life that you live.

On a positive note you don't have to change all of those thoughts to bring about positive change in you life. It is estimated that we need to direct just 1,000 to 2,000 of our daily thoughts on a new goal to make it a reality, because wherever your attention goes, the energy flows. What your mind focuses on in life is what you get back.

Here is a simple exercise to demonstrate that what you focus on becomes your reality.

Exercise #19:
The Power Of Your Attention

Bring your attention to your right thumb, look at it, sense it, feel it, study your right thumb without judgment, completely absorb yourself in its detail. Your thumb is all that exists for you right now. Now notice how much you appreciate your thumb, how much it does for you without you even knowing or being aware of it. How much a vital part of yourself it is. Your thumb is tiny, but notice how nothing else exists except your thumb as you focus on it. Your thumb is everything in this moment, nothing else exists.

Next, read through the following exercise then close your eyes and bring your focus internally to something in your life that irritates or upsets you. How does this something make you feel? Completely submerge yourself in this feeling. Notice where you feel it in your body. Notice your breathing, notice your heart rate and observe all your thoughts about this thing. Notice how the thoughts and stories you now have about this issue have momentum of their own, like the car rolling down a hill. This problem is really real for you right now and your body believes it.

Notice that you have brought your upset about this issue into this present moment and because of your focus on it, it feels really real to you now. Because it feels real, it has become fixed and it has become a belief. Through your thoughts, you have manifested it and magnified it and your body believes it to be real and to be happening now. Your own thoughts have increased your heart rate, and this issue appears to be getting bigger and bigger because you are focusing on it.

Now open your eyes and go back to the study of your thumb, completely absorb yourself in the focus of your thumb. What exists for you now? Is your previous concern beginning to disappear as you bring your attention back into the present moment? Breathe in deeply and bring your focus back to now, to your body, to the present moment.

What you think of, you will get more of it. If your focus is on negative thoughts you will fill your MindBody with negative thinking. If you keep bringing your awareness to the beauty of the present moment by connecting to your body, you will fill your MindBody with positive thinking. From this space you can begin to focus on generating more thoughts about what you do want from life and let go of obsessive thinking about the things you don't want.

This is how awesomely powerful you are! If you hold onto a thought it will grow and become real. For example, if a superstitious person walks under a ladder and believes it will bring him bad luck, then it probably will. Carrying a lucky talisman will bring you luck, but only if you believe it will. This is the power of your own mind. Belief creates your experiences and not vice versa! If you want to change your circumstances in life, then you must change your beliefs about those circumstances first.

As the inspirational Dr Wayne Dyer once said, 'When you change the way you look at things, things you look at change'.

To truly empower yourself is to understand that the primary cause of any unhappiness you have in your life is never actually about the situation, but about the thoughts you have about the situation and how you allow it to affect you. What do you make these experiences mean? What is your belief about it? Do you make it mean you are worthless? Penniless? Unlucky? A failure? A bad mother, father or lover?

These are all just labels you have made up about yourself that become true because you believe it! To become a master over your thoughts is to become the observer of your thoughts, and not to become your thoughts! Happiness is a decision not a condition and it's a decision that only you can make for yourself, nobody else can.

Mind Your Words

Your word has tremendous power. Whenever you say anything, you are literally giving your word. The energy of your intention behind the word is also truly powerful. Your words come from your thoughts and your thoughts come mostly from a pre-programmed positive or negative response within you. Do you more often say, "I can', or do you say, 'I can't'. Either one will come true for you.

What are your daily affirmations you use that create your life?

A woman I know uses the same affirmation every time I see her. She says, 'Sod's Law!', which means "if something can go wrong, then it will". Every time she says 'Sod's Law!' she is affirming her belief that things always go wrong for her. And because she says 'Sod's Law' day in day out, guess what happens? She constantly has the experience of things going wrong in her life.

In its own right, the phrase 'Sod's Law!' is meaningless, but to the woman whose mantra it is, the phrase affirms a deeply held belief that she has cultivated over the years that things always go wrong. All of us have habitual thoughts like this that aren't real. It's easy to spot other people's, but it takes real mastery to spot our own negative mantras and beliefs and begin to interrupt these thought patterns and create new, resourceful affirmations for ourselves.

Over the years I've collected stories from people who manifest what they don't want. Like the woman whose unconscious catchphrase was 'that's the trouble you see', who experienced life as being filled with trouble, every single day. Or the man who was shortsighted who kept losing his glasses and kept saying, 'I wish I didn't have to wear my glasses'. What he really wanted was perfect eyesight, but all his unconscious heard was his impatient desire to rid him of wearing glasses, hence the constant disappearance of them! Then there was a wealthy woman who just wanted a simple life and kept saying, 'I wish I lived in a shed!'. Eventually through unfortunate circumstances she lost all her money and she did in fact end up living in a shed!

So as the old adage goes, be careful what you wish for, because it might come true.

One way to discover what affirmations or words you are unconsciously using to create your life circumstances, is to ask a close friend or a family member (as we often don't notice our mantras until someone else points them out).

What word or phrase have you discovered that you use a lot? You may find clues in the words you have written down during the exercises in this book. What word or phrase pops up regularly? Have you noticed how this word or phrase seems to bring more of that word in to your life? For example, if you use the word 'love' a lot in your life, then you will attract love. If you use the word 'hate' regularly, then you will attract hate.

There is an amazing book written by a Japanese scientist called Dr Masaru Emoto called 'The hidden messages in water'. In this book he reveals the effects of how our words, thoughts and emotions have on physical matter. Dr Emoto takes high speed photographs of frozen water to reveal how the crystals formed in the water (before it's frozen) change when specific concentrated thoughts and words are directed towards them. The water that has been exposed to loving, positive words, show brilliant complex snowflake patterns and in contrast, water exposed to negative hateful thoughts, form incomplete asymmetrical patterns which are dull or black in colour. Since these findings by Masaru Emoto, this kind of experiment has been repeated many times by many people to prove that positive and negative words have a profound and lasting effect on life forms.

You can try a simpler experiment yourself. Find two identical plants and put them near to each other but not too close together. To one of the plants speak negative nasty words to it every day for three weeks. To the other plant only send loving positive words to it every day for three weeks. After the third week notice the difference in the plants. The one that had loving thoughts directed to it will be healthy and growing rapidly, the one you directed nasty negative words to will look diseased and unhealthy.

Another experiment you can try is with rice. Get two jam jars and fill them a quarter full with rice and then half fill the jars with water. Put a label on one saying 'I hate you' and put a label on the other saying, 'I love you', Do the same as you did with the plant experiment, spend three weeks sending nasty negative words to the one labelled 'I hate you' and loving positive words to the other.

After three weeks you will notice the rice that had positive words directed to it had not changed, yet the rice that had negative words directed to it will be mouldy. This is the result of human thoughts, intention and the spoken word. Considering we are almost 90% water, can you imagine what effect we have on ourselves and others when we think or speak negative words! It is easy to continue with our old habits of thinking, but if you do nothing to change your negative thoughts, then nothing will change. Your health, your relationships, your finances, your life, will all stay the same and may get worse.

What do your words keep attracting to you in life? What goes on in your head? What self-talk do you use? How do you see the world? What changes can you personally make to stop repeated patterns? It starts by changing your mind and also your beliefs.

The Power Of Self-Belief

Beliefs originate from our parents, our social conditioning and our culture. We inherit beliefs without questioning them and accept that they are true. We live our lives by our beliefs. Our beliefs control our biology. We usually believe something to be true until it is proven otherwise. Just like humans believed the world was flat until it was proven to be round. Our beliefs are locked into place by the beliefs of those around us and it takes a lot of conscious effort and our own inner convictions to change a collective belief.

If we believe something to be true, it can become true. The great example is the four minute mile. It was first achieved in 1954 by Roger Bannister and before that nobody thought it was possible and because no one thought it possible, no one achieved it. As soon as Roger proved he could run a mile in four minutes, suddenly lots of people could do it. The reason is because their belief about what was possible changed.

Henry Ford, the great automobile manufacturer said, 'Whether you believe you can, or whether you believe you can't, you're right'. We set our own limit on what we believe to be possible. Beliefs are very powerful and when we focus on something we give it energy and momentum, just like taking the brakes off a car at the top of a hill. The momentum gets greater and it can't be stopped. This is the same with your thoughts.

Apparently it takes just 17 seconds of any thought, be it positive or negative to draw another positive or negative thought to you. If you think negatively for 1 minute, then it's really difficult to shift out of that train of thought again. It carves a groove of thought, like the constant dripping of rain that eventually creates a stream. If you think a thought enough it turns into a belief. A belief is just a thought you continually think. We like to label things, name them, and when we label and name something, it becomes real and fixed. It turns into a belief. It isn't necessarily true, but we believe it to be true even though we made it up in the first place!

Are any of these statements your beliefs? 'Old age brings illness'; 'No pain no gain'; I'm always unlucky'; 'Stress can kill you'; You just can't win'; 'Good things always come to an end'; 'Revenge is sweet'; 'I'm no good with finances'; 'Love doesn't last'; 'I'm hopeless/stupid/unhealthy/unlucky in love'; 'If I imagine the worst that can happen, then I won't be disappointed when it does'; 'I have to be perfect to be loved'; I'm unlovable'; 'I never get it right'; You can't trust anyone', 'I never have time'.

Whatever you focus on, you get more of. Focus on agitation, you get more agitation. Focus on the good stuff in your life, you get more good stuff. Focus on your bad health, you get more bad health. Focus on love, you get more love.

If you have people in your life that set off your stress responses, then it is an indication that you have an unconscious negative belief system linked to that relationship. No one can 'push your buttons' (triggering your stress response) unless you have belief patterns and old programming that needs to be healed.

For instance, Frank had a mother who was very protective towards him, to the extent of being jealous of any girl he would bring home. Frank couldn't bare his mother's smothering attitude and so left home as soon as he was old enough to do so. Soon after he met a woman and moved in with her, only to find she was exactly like his mother, smothering and possessive. So by moving away from his mother, he realised that he'd actually moved back in with her! He kept moving from one girlfriend to the next, but found the same pattern kept being repeated. Why is this? His neural pathways had been programmed to believe that his mother's over protection and smothering represented love.

We often attract to us people with the same energy patterning as our own. We attract people to us that 'feel right' to us, mirroring our own programming. We associate dependency and familiarity with love. If you associate love with shame, guilt, abandonment, loss, disapproval, pain or abuse, then you are unlikely to find a harmonious relationship, because you will be attracting to you someone with similar beliefs as yours.

Another common problem is if you had a troubled childhood, then you will have built up a concoction of defence strategies to help you cope, which will play out in your current relationships, so the wheel of destruction will just keep turning until the program or belief patterning has been changed.

If you cannot love yourself, but need the love of others to fulfil you, then you will be in a relationship based on needs. If you seek approval and ignore your own needs, or if you settle for second best, blame others, ignore your dreams, then you will be operating from your insecurity and you are more likely to attract someone who is also insecure.

The best way to tackle any unharmonious relationships, is honesty. Be honest with yourself and others rather than hiding behind guilt and shame. When you are honest in relationships, and uncover your underlying belief system around love and intimacy, then the relationship will move to a new level. When you are authentic, your relationships become authentic and this is the perfect condition for all wounded parties to repair their old wounds and heal. Once you have embraced, learnt and healed old belief systems and energetic patterns, then you can move on to a new positive future.

What's Your Core Belief System?

Now you have begun to realise how powerful your mind is and how it directs your life. You may have discovered some of your unconscious programming which dictates your patterns and your life. You may have discovered that the choices and decisions you make are decided by your programming instead of your true self and true feelings. You have discovered that you create your world and what shows up in it and that the thoughts you think and the words you use, create your world. You now know that by changing your old thoughts, habits and emotional responses with conscious practice, you will change your life experiences. And with patience and conscious practice, you now know that you can rewire your unconscious reactive patterns into new thoughts and reactions that will bring you health and happiness.

To rewire your patterns and reactions you first need to discover the primary unconscious programming that's running your life. What main belief system is steering your ship? It is time to take a closer look at the words and notes you have written down throughout this book to find your primary unconscious belief. Keep your notes safe as you will need them again at the end of this book.

Firstly, look at your notes to find what area of your body and which body centre is the most blocked or out of balance. Is it your moving centre (hips downwards) which relate to your stability and direction? Your being centre (back and torso) which relates to your self-esteem, personal power and self-acceptance? Your doing centre (your shoulders and arms) which relate to your ability to give and receive, and to physically express yourself? Your control centre (your head, neck, face) which relates to a need to be in control? You may have a few problem areas which are not in just one body centre. What thoughts did you write down about these areas? Do you physically have any problems or health issues in these areas? Do you see any connection between your thoughts and your physical issues?

Now, look at all the words and the notes you have written down for all of your body centres throughout reading this book. All the words you have written are telling you about you, about what you feel and who you are right now. This is the self-talk which is running your life. Is there an overall theme or story of self-talk running through each exercise? Is there a main word or phrase that keeps cropping up? What is this word or phrase? Is there a story emerging? What is your story? Is it a positive or negative story? What is the mantra you use that creates your life experiences and your limitations?

If you found you wrote down mainly negative or destructive words or phrases, then it is time to find the root cause of these negative words you use that shapes your body and your life.

Write a phrase about your main theme or 'story' about you and your life, with the words you have written and the realisations you have discovered throughout the book. This way you will get a clear picture of what is responsible for your health and your life patterns.

You will need to remember your main word, phrase or sentence in the next meditation.

♥ Meditation #8: Clear Your Mind

Allow 20 minutes for this meditation. Read through it first or get someone to read it to you. Get into a comfortable position and close your eyes. Take some deep breaths and allow your body to relax. To clear your mind, imagine you are a little being in your mind who has a broom. Imagine yourself sweeping your thoughts away. Sweep into every corner of your mind until it is clean and clear. You might even want to use an imaginary vacuum cleaner to suck out the thoughts that are particularly stubborn! Once your mind is clear and your body is relaxed, place your word or phrase into the clear space of your mind. Start to feel what this word or phrase really means to you. Start to feel the words as an emotion. How does this words or phrase make you feel?

Does this word, phrase or feeling relate to your present life situation or circumstances? Have you ever felt this feeling before? If so when? Can you relate it to any feelings from a past situation? Any memory that comes to mind? Allow your unconscious to talk to you. Allow any past memory or feeling to be heard. It wants to be acknowledged.

If a memory came up which is related to your word or phrase, allow the feeling attached to the memory to expand. Welcome the feeling. Notice where in your body you feel it the most. Allow it to be expressed. Keep expanding the feeling no matter how uncomfortable and unpleasant it feels. It wants expression and it wants to be heard. Let your emotions surface, feel the liberation of the emotions as they rise, fully feel the emotion. Now lovingly tell this part of you that you are safe and it is now time to let the memory heal. It is now time to let it go. So take a deep breath into your tummy and with the out breath, release the memory or feeling. And another breath in and push it out of your body with the out breath. One more breath and it has now gone.

Now start to breathe love into your belly. Like you would love a child or a loved one. Breathe in love from your heart and direct it into your belly, then to the area you felt emotion and then to the rest of your body. Breathe in loving light and allow any remaining blocks and stuck energy to dissolve. Keep breathing and releasing.

One more breath and with the out breath let any tension in your body go. Let it go. All fears related to this memory have now dissolved. It is now no longer a part of you. Feel how clear and free your mind and body is now.

The Tale Of The Father Who Couldn't Let Go

Being brave enough to change your patterns and beliefs requires taking a few committed steps. One of my clients, Christine, initially came to see me for a sports massage because her hip and shoulder hurt. I treated her symptoms in the way a sports massage therapist is trained, but I couldn't help but get an overwhelming feeling that Christine's problems went beyond the physical (as they nearly always do) and that the massage wasn't really making a difference.

To me her whole body screamed 'stuck' and 'blocked' and no matter how much I pummelled her, I didn't think it was helping. I didn't know how she would feel if I shared this information with her, but my intuition told me it was okay. Once I told her what I picked up from her during her treatment, she looked at me with an ashen face and said she felt so depressed and 'stuck' in her life and she didn't know what to do!

Christine then became a regular client of mine. We worked through all the blocks that she had unconsciously created in her life which included her work (as a teacher) her relationship with her ex-husband, her aching body and her weight issues. Her hips represented feeling stuck in her career and her creativity and her shoulders represented the load she was carrying, particularly with her pupils and a sick father.

Over the period of a year we worked on these issues through body work, healing, positive affirmations and MindBody reprogramming. Christine also attended my MindBody Journey course. After a year, the difference in Christine was profound and, as she said, in her own words, 'I feel like a new woman'. Her hip and shoulder pain had gone, she had left her job and moved away to an area that suited her better, she lost lots of weight and she started dating again after 12 years of being single. Needless to say she was a very happy woman and was no longer 'stuck'.

But one thing still bothered her and that was her father. He was ill with cancer and had been for over six years. She drove 50 miles every week to be with him, but she never felt she had his love or approval. Once she was totally honest about her feelings, she realised that she felt that he was 'hanging on' and wouldn't let her go just to spite her. She just wanted him to pass away so she could be free! Free from the pain she felt from his disapproval and his disappointment of her. She felt that her father was blocking her freedom to be herself. So during one session we decided to heal this issue she had with her father once and for all.

I asked her questions about how she felt about her father. One thing that was loud and clear, was that she was angry with him. She felt she had never been respected, never allowed to make her own decisions and that she always felt judged by him. Because these beliefs were so strong in her MindBody (being disrespected, disapproved of and being judged) she attracted relationships into her life that mirrored these beliefs.

I asked her 'Are you ready to drop this belief system?' She replied 'Yes'. I then asked, 'Are you ready to set your father free?' She said yes but it was a hesitant yes, so I repeated the question until she fully felt it within her body and until her 'Yes' was strong and definite. We then did a healing and a meditation to finally release this old programming.

It wasn't her father who couldn't let go of her and set her free like she believed, it was the other way round. She could not let go of her father because of what she believed he thought about her. She couldn't forgive him. Once she realised it was her that was holding him back, that it was her beliefs and her upset, not his, was she able to let him go. He was not to blame. He loved her and was just being himself with all his unhealthy programming and belief systems. She finally forgave her father and three days after this healing session, Christine's father passed away. She had finally set HIM free!!

KEY LESSONS FROM CHAPTER FOURTEEN

• Beliefs are not real, they are just thoughts that you habitually think

• Your beliefs about the world are revealed in the repeated thoughts you think, the words you speak and the emotions you feel

• Your thoughts, words and emotions are daily affirmations that shape the life you live

CHAPTER FIFTEEN

Connecting To Your Soul

Before you get to the final completion stage of Your MindBody Journey, where you will be reprogramming your MindBody 'story' and negative belief systems, I would like to invite you to consider the bigger picture.

The purpose of this book has been to take you on a personal journey of discovery to explore what your body can reveal about your mind. Yet at some level you already know that there is more to you than just your MindBody. There is a part of you that lives both within you and beyond the limits of your body that we refer to as your soul.

Your mind, body and soul are not separate but they operate as one unit. If your body is sick, it's because your mind is sick and your mind is sick because your soul is sick. What does this mean? It means that if one part of you suffers, they all suffer and mostly the suffering originates from your deepest place, your soul.

You may ask questions like, 'Who am I?'; 'What is my soul?'; 'Where does my soul live?'

Your soul is already there within you. You will find it beyond your mind and your body. Your soul is both within you and beyond you as it's not restricted by physical boundaries. Your soul is beyond the labels you have for yourself like mother/father; sister/brother; son/daughter; husband/wife; partner/friend; the title you have at work or the person you are at parties. Your soul is not the 'story' you like to tell the world about who you are, that is your persona. Your soul is the deeper part of you beyond what your mind thinks and beyond the emotions you feel. It's beyond your ego, your persona, your hurts, your pains and your past. It is the still, wise, all knowing, all loving part of you. It is the you that shows up when you are still and quiet, when your thoughts and feelings are absent. It is your essence, your inner knowing, your unique energy that survives beyond physical death. When you operate from your soul as opposed to your mind, the selfish part of you disappears, you are happy to serve unconditionally rather than wanting a payback whenever you give out. Everything vibrates at a certain frequency and creates a forcefield around it. This is your aura. And because we are magnetic beings and vibrate at a certain frequency, we can magnetise whatever we truly want and need in life when we are connected to our soul's purpose.

When you are not in alignment or connected with your soul, struggle begins and your emotional and physical health suffers. When you are in alignment and are in harmony with your soul, things in life flow easily and effortlessly and the natural outcome is happiness, health and vitality.

Exercise #20:
Mastering Stillness

Take a moment to be still and quiet. Take some deep breaths and allow the constant flow of thoughts to float by and drift away so your mind is still. Like shaking a jar of muddy water, it takes a while for the grains of soil to settle at the bottom of the jar and for the clear water to emerge. Have patience with yourself knowing there are such depths of pleasures to discover once you have mastered the constant chatter of your thoughts.

Once you have mastered the stillness within you, open yourself up to a wider space of nothingness. Keep expanding into the nothingness until you feel a wealth of 'everything-ness' a richness and clarity where time does not exist. Soon you will be feeling a sensation of love and bliss. This make take practice and patience to achieve or it may take you only a few moments. Everyone is different.

When you have reached the place of infinite love within you, you are now with the 'oneness', the 'universe', 'the divine' the 'universal intelligence', higher consciousness', the 'field', 'spirit' or 'god' whatever label you want to give it. This is your true essence, it is yours, it is you, it is your soul and it is always there with you and always will be!

Realms Of Consciousness

Through a microscope we can now see life forms that we previously had no idea existed, they were not in our realm of consciousness. Life forms exist even beyond the microscope, so small that no instrument we have designed can ever detect them. This doesn't mean they don't exist, just that they live beyond the limits of human detection. In fact, microscopic life forms are infinitesimal, meaning there is no end of things getting smaller. The same is true regarding the macrocosm. Things exist beyond our realm of existence, and there is no end to infinite nature of the cosmos, just because the strongest telescopes can't see something, doesn't mean they don't exist. Electricity exists, but because we can't see it, it doesn't mean it doesn't exist. Other forms of life exist, just because they are not observable or measurable in our realm of consciousness, doesn't mean they don't exist.

To understand this better, consider the natural world. A fish that swims in the sea has no idea that grass exists, it doesn't mean that grass doesn't exist just because it's not in the realm of consciousness of the fish. A bee, worm or ant has no awareness of our human existence, it isn't in their realm of consciousness, but it is a fact that we do exist, just not to them. The same can be said about human existence. A rabbit in a cage only knows the reality of its cage, it doesn't have any consciousness to understand that there are cities beyond it, countries even, planets even, universes even! We are the same as the rabbit in its cage, we are limited by our perceptions and our own environment.

Other things exist beyond us that we have no way of detecting, like a higher consciousness and a higher intelligence. I won't use the word God to describe this as the concept of God has become divisive and distorted, especially through religion, so I will use the word 'the greater consciousness' instead. This greater consciousness is forever expanding and never ending. Just like the universe, the universe never ends, it is constantly expanding, and we expand with it. It is not linear, it has no end or beginning, it is holographic. Nothing is fixed, there is no truth, because the truth keeps changing and evolving through expansion, something our limited brains have difficulty grasping. We are all part of this evolution, and we are growing and evolving into a new realm of existence, whether we like it or not.

Whichever way we want to view life, if we evolve with ease and acceptance, we don't go through growing pains, we will evolve and grow effortlessly, but if we resist change and evolution, then we will struggle.

Choosing Your Frequency

Like everything in the universe, we are made of energy and energy cannot disappear, it transforms into something else. When ice melts it becomes water and when water heats up it becomes steam. Clouds become rain and raindrops become streams and rivers and waves, and great oceans freeze and become great icebergs. Like water, energy cannot disappear and because we are energy, we do not disappear once we die just because we've lost our bodies, we instead evolve into a new form.

When we fully understand that we are part of the collective oneness, we are the drop that makes up the ocean, we are the blade of grass that makes the meadow, we are the leaves that make the tree, we are part of the great cosmic intelligence, we are not separate, we are all one so therefore we are part of the greater consciousness. Then we will realise that we are capable of anything and everything.

Being part of the collective oneness is a difficult concept to grasp for most people because we feel so separate. We believe we are on this planet alone, our thoughts and feelings are exclusive only to us, but believe it or not, everyone feels and thinks the same to some degree. This is because we are part of the collective consciousness, which we tap into via our energetic system, therefore we are all one. All plants, animals, rocks and all living things vibrate at a certain electromagnetic frequency and so all things are connected and interrelated.

The famous story of the 100th monkey helps illustrates this point. In 1952 a group of Scientists were studying the Macaque monkey on the Japanese Island of Koshima. These monkeys used to feed on sweet potatoes, which they loved, but they didn't like the taste of the dirt on the potatoes. One day, one of the monkeys discovered that if it washed the sweet potatoes in water, especially salt water, they would taste better. Soon the technique was copied by other members of the monkey family, each monkey copying the other. The knowledge spread and soon nearly all the monkeys on the island were using the same technique. It is said that when the 100th monkey learnt this technique, something remarkable happened. The knowledge hopped over the sea and soon all the Macaque monkeys on the neighbouring islands were washing sweet potatoes in water too! How did this information get across a wide expanse of water? This is the power of the collective unconscious in action.

We are tapping into this big pool of collective unconscious all the time, picking up knowledge, information and emotions without even realising it. Most of the time we unconsciously choose to tap into a particular range of thought or emotions within the big pool of consciousness, a bit like tuning into a particular frequency on a radio station.

If we tune into 'Happiness FM', for example, then we get happiness. If we decide to tune into 'Sadness FM' then we get sadness. They are many different emotional frequencies ranging from the lowest (fear) and the highest (love) and thousands of frequencies in-between: resentment, jealousy, gratitude, empathy etc. Sometimes we get stuck on one channel and only want to listen to 'Radio Resentment', for example, and that's why we feel resentment all the time and keep manifesting more things to feel resentful about. If we consciously choose to change the station, to tune into a different emotional channel, such as 'Forgiveness FM', then we will experience forgiveness.

I know, from personal experience, that tuning into a different frequency is sometimes easier said than done, especially when our programming is so strong, the tuning buttons might be a little stuck! But with conscious practice, patience and perseverance, you can and will change.

Faith And Trust

When we trust in our higher power and know that we are connected to a greater consciousness, then our struggles disappear. We are not alone, never were and never will be. Inside of you is the same intelligence that holds the universe in place, the same intelligence that tells the chick when to crack open its egg, the same intelligence that tells the rose bud when to open. The famous author Anaïs Nin wrote beautifully, 'the risk in keeping your rose bud tight is more painful than the risk to blossom'. The divine wisdom within you knows you must open and blossom. The pain we suffer is only because we resist.

If life gets really tough and we have tried everything we can to take responsibility for our issues and have done all we can by changing our habits, patterns and negative thoughts to resolve our inner conflicts, then we sometimes need to just surrender, to 'let go and let God'. Some things are just meant to be.

The Tale Of A Truly Beautiful Woman

Many years ago, I was fortunate enough to treat one of the most inspiring and beautiful women I have ever met.

When I first opened the door to her, my jaw hit the floor. Quickly recovering myself so as not to let her see my response, I invited her in with a smile. She looked like a female version of the elephant man, this is the only way I could describe her. Where her ears and eyes used to be there were just holes and she had painted eyelashes and eyebrows with an eyeliner pencil to represent her eyes. Where her fingers used to be there were just stumps. She had painted red nail vanish on her stumps to represent her toes and fingers. Where her hair used to be, there was a long blond wig. Her speech was slow and rasping. I swallowed hard as a sympathetic lump formed in my throat for this poor woman.

Once she was on the couch and I started her treatment, she told me her story. She used to be a fashion model for beauty products and swimwear until one day she was trapped in a house fire. Luckily she survived, but as a result she was severely disfigured. It took her ten long years to get from a place of anger, blame, grief, pain and non-acceptance of her condition, to a place of acceptance and love for herself and for who she had become.

Because she was such a beauty before the fire, she had been on a long journey from hating her appearance and not accepting what had happened to her and her career, to deep soul searching which lead her to finally loving and accepting who she was regardless of her disfigurement. Because she could finally accept and love who she was now, physically, mentally and spiritually, she received deep love and acceptance back.

After the treatment it was so beautiful to watch as she smoothed down her false hair with love and pride, how she reapplied her make up with care and attention, how she held her head high and mostly how she was so open and loving. She was truly an inspiration and it put my petty concerns to shame.

Learning to love yourself, warts and all, no matter what, is the quickest route to experiencing unconditional love for yourself and from others. By learning to trust your path, accepting what shows up along the way and going with the universal flow of life, you learn faith.

Believe In Your Self

When you have a solid, undoubting belief in yourself and your path, you have faith. When you have an unwavering faith that everything will be okay (whatever that may mean for you), and when you have faced your own resistance and shifted from believing something is not right in your life to believing anything you want to achieve is possible, it allows miracles to happen. When all doubts have been removed and resistance has gone, anything can happen. Your electromagnetic force field can then draw the future to you.

This wisdom has been passed on to use through the ages by spiritual masters like Buddha, Jesus and Ghandi. They have all passed this knowledge of faith and trust to us. When you believe in your higher power (which is the same as their power) and you trust that you are a part of an almighty consciousness, and when you have unwavering faith and trust, mountains move and magic happens.

The Tale Of The Lost Traveller

I remember once visiting New York as a young adult, walking down a street unsure of where I was heading. The further I went, the more unsure I became, until it dawned on me that I was completely and utterly lost! Being a tourist I felt very vulnerable and a fear and panic started to kick in. This was before the days of GPS and mobile phones and so I felt so lost, alone and scared, desperately searching a friendly face to ask directions.

It was then I had a good talk with myself and reminded myself of the power of my own mind and my connection to the universal consciousness. If I believed I was lost, then I was. So I changed my belief system to 'I know exactly where I am and I am always guided'. At that very moment something fluttered past my feet. Initially I thought it was a piece of rubbish, but as I looked closer my heart filled with wonder and joy as I realised what it was. I bent down and picked it up and in my hand I had a detailed tourist street map of New York that someone must have dropped or thrown away!!

I said a HUGE thank you and with a big smile on my face I found my bearings and set back on the right path. I see this as an analogy for life. When we get lost in life and are fearful of our future and direction, all we have to do is let go of our fears and affirm that we are always guided to be exactly where we need to be, then a map will always appear, in whatever form that is, to help us find our way.

Healing The Wounded Soul

If you have deep-rooted pain, simply changing the way you think or having faith, can sometimes take a long time to heal the pain and suffering held within your energy field. If you've had a traumatic or painful past, then deeper healing may be needed. There is a lot of help available in the form of counselling, trauma therapy, support groups, body work, hands on healing and even past-life regression and it is good to pick whatever therapy you feel drawn to. Everyone is different and every pain is different, use your intuition to guide you.

To complicate matters further, we sometimes hold on to pain and suffering from our ancestors, which has been passed down the family line in our DNA without us even knowing about it! If you think this might be the case for you, that there seems to be a repeated pattern in your ancestral past which is similar to your own, then with intention you can let go of this past pattern of suffering.

This can be done in a number of ways. You can cut the energetic chords that tie you to the past in a visualisation or meditation; you can say a decree out loud three times, asking for the past suffering to end here and now; you can visualise your DNA, reprogramming the past pattern and create a new pattern that serves you and the life you want to live. It is best to find a reputable healer or therapist to help you with this and again use your intuition to find the right one for you.

I believe that bad things 'happen' to us because we have not yet healed, haven't forgiven or are holding on to a belief that no longer serves us. Sometimes just to understand 'why' something has 'happened' to us can lessen the trauma.

I believe there are no coincidences and we are on a unique journey of learning and sometimes the tougher the lessons and the bigger the trauma, the greater the opportunity for growth and learning there is for us. Sometimes we have to learn the hard way by experiencing unpleasant things for our unresolved issues to come to the surface and be healed. If you haven't released, forgiven or healed a past pain or trauma, but continue to hold on to it, then it will eventually show up in your present life, either through a similar experience or through your body in the form of dis-ease. This doesn't happen to torture or punish us, but to guide us to live happier, healthier lives.

The Tale Of Healing And Empowerment

I had an experience when I was 36 which I didn't think I would ever get over, but I believe it had to happen because I was ignoring and burying a past pain deep within me. I will share my story, however it may be a little disturbing or upsetting for some.

I was on a beach near to where I lived in Australia at the time and had just been for a swim and settled myself in the sand dunes to dry off before heading back home. Suddenly, from behind the sand dunes, a man appeared wearing a balaclava to hide his face.

He was holding a shotgun.

He proved to me the shotgun was loaded and he wasn't afraid of using it. He pounced on top of me and with one of his hands pointed the gun in my back, with the other hand he tried to handcuff me. He clearly intended to rape me and I was petrified. My natural fight, flight or freeze mechanisms kicked in and luckily I didn't freeze, I fought! I struggled and squirmed under his weight and he was yelling, 'I'll kill you if you don't lay still'.

Suddenly from nowhere, I had an overwhelming will and conviction rise within me. I realised that I wasn't afraid of death, but I was afraid of rape. So I said to him, 'You can kill me, but you are NOT going to rape me!' He dropped the gun so he could then use both hands to try again to handcuff me. My will, inner power and conviction was so strong that with all his strength (and he was a big man) he couldn't hold me down. I managed to pull myself up, he dived on me and pulled me back down again. 'Why was there no one else on the beach?' I thought. I was in this on my own. This wrestling went on for what seemed like forever, I'd make a dash for it and then he would jump back on top of me again. He then dragged me into the bush behind the dunes and at that point I knew it was the point of no return, this was it, I was about to be raped.

It was then that I let go and let God. I surrendered and trusted and it was at that point when I saw a figure on the beach in the distance. I managed to release one arm from his grip and I waved and I yelled 'Help me! Help me!'. At that point my attacker realised we weren't alone and let me go. I fled in one direction and he ran off in the other.

I ran for help and the police were called. It seemed like a happy ending, but the big ordeal didn't stop there. A long extensive search went on to find the attacker, but he was never found. This left me with an absolute feeling of terror with constant questions running round and round in my head. 'What if it's someone who knows me?'; 'What if he's a neighbour and follows me?' 'He's out there somewhere, what if he tries to do it again?'.

I got to the point where I was too scared to leave the house. I became agoraphobic. The slightest sounds made me jump in hysteria. When I did occasionally find the courage to go outside, any male presence used to freak me out. 'It could be him!' I kept chanting. I was damaged, not physically, but emotionally. Emotional damage can take a long time to heal and can even stay with us forever. The worst part about the whole of the experience for me, was that the attacker had taken away my freedom. I no longer felt free to go where I wanted and I no longer trusted men. I was a changed, damaged woman and I hated that the most.

It was after about six months that I realised I couldn't go on feeling this way any longer. I wanted to get my life back and my freedom and power. I believed HE had taken my power away. But in fact I had taken my own power away. I believed all men were potential rapists and I believed I was now never safe. The type of experience I had, being attacked by a stranger in a public place, is extremely rare but I believed it could happen again at any time. I was tormenting myself and I knew this had to stop. So one day, I drew upon all my inner power to get myself back out there alone again. I used all my inner strength to walk along the beach every day where the attack happened to build up my confidence, and I then used all my courage to get help in the form of counselling and healing.

Looking back, I can now honestly say the attack was one of the best things that had happened to me. This might sound like an odd thing to say, but what it did was bring up all my hidden issues and made me face them. My hidden issues were the very things that stopped me fulfilling my potential in my relationships, my work, my life. I had been stuck for a long time, not really knowing why. I kept repeating the same disastrous patterns one after the other. I went through one relationship after the other, never staying put for long. I didn't realise it until the counselling that I had an issue with men even before the attack happened.

All my life I had kept a secret of an incident that had happened to me when I was 11 years old. I was sexually assaulted by a stranger in the woods near to where I lived in England and I had pushed the memory deep inside of me to a place where it could never hurt me. However my subconscious was running a different set of rules. It was running the programming of 'all males are potential rapists', and that, 'men are never to be trusted' and that 'sex was abusive'.

This programming played out throughout all my adult relationships and I couldn't understand why I was so unsuccessful in love. I craved love, but I was too scared to surrender myself fully to it, always keeping people at arms length. I had such a deep male issue and an issue with sex, that no wonder it never worked out. I also had physical symptoms that corresponded to my beliefs. I used to suffer from severe period pains, endometriosis, kidney infections and psoriasis around my pubic bone. This, I now realise, was due to a blocked sacral chakra, which governs the sexual organs and glands and our ability for healthy relationships.

Through counselling, the memory of my childhood assault had to come to the surface to be healed. I had to change the inner dialogue that I had about men and I had to rewire my programming with a more positive story.

After a lot of work and perseverance it payed off. A deep healing went on inside me. I forgave my attacker, knowing he was obviously deep in pain himself to do such a thing, or had such low self esteem that he couldn't interact healthily with women. I finally learnt to trust men, to love the masculine energy within myself and cherish my relationships with the men in my life. Because I had changed my belief from 'all men are bastards' to 'all men are loving and kind', this is what I finally attracted. I am now in a very loving and fulfilling relationship with a beautiful and kind man who is my life partner. My health issues connected to my sacral chakra also disappeared.

♥ Meditation #9: Healing Deep Wounds

Here is a guided meditation that will help you to heal any deep wounds you may have within your soul memory. Read it first or get someone to read it out to you. Allow about 15-20 minutes. Repeat this meditation as often as you feel you need to.

Make sure your body is in a comfortable position and make sure you won't be disturbed.

Take in some deep breaths and allow your body to relax. Keep your focus on your deep breathing until your mind and body are still and peaceful. In your mind's eye you see in front of you a beautiful temple or building. You sense that this temple is a very special place of healing. There is a path that leads up to the temple and you feel drawn to walk up the path until you get to the temple door. You see your name is written on the front of the door and the door slowly opens. You are greeted by a great wise being. It may be one of your past ancestors, Ghandi, Buddha, an angel, someone you admire and trust, whatever you feel comfortable with. They greet you with such warmth and love and you feel your body relax. Your inner knowing knows you trust this person, they are there to help you and to help your soul to heal.

They guide you into the temple and you take a while to look around you. You absorb its splendour and beauty. There are beautiful colours, like rainbows dancing across the walls. You know this is a very special place and it is there just for you. In the centre of this temple you see a big column of bright light shafting down from the ceiling onto the floor below. You are drawn to go to this light and the wise being encourages you forward towards this beam of light. The light is like nothing you have ever seen, so warm, sparkly and bright, but it isn't a brightness that makes you close your eyes, it's a brightness that opens your eyes (and your heart and mind too).

You now step under this light and instantly you feel this brilliant light cleansing you. You feel it cleansing and activating every one of your chakras. The light travels down your spine, penetrating through the top of your head, into the middle of your brain, down to your neck, to your heart, through your tummy, your hips, the base of your spine and down your legs and out through your feet. You feel this light changing the form of your DNA.

This light is reprogramming your pain that has been held within your cells and is clearing all your unresolved emotional wounds. Your cells that hold the old memory are starting to change. You can feel your cells transforming from a dark colour to bright light. The light has activated your DNA to a new healthy patterning and created a new blueprint for your future. The column of light cleanses your entire being, not just your physical body, but your energy body, your chakras and your aura. Like a waterfall of light surging through your entire being. You feel your whole body radiate with light. Bathe in this light for as long as you feel you need to, then when you are ready, step out of the light where your wise guide is waiting for you.

Your guide is smiling at you knowing all your pains and wounds have now been dissolved. Your guide pours unconditional love into you from their open heart and you return this unconditional love back. You feel filled with love and lightness. Your wise person leans towards you and whispers in your ear a final piece of guidance that is important for you. Be receptive and listen until you hear your guidance.

You are then guided back to the door of the temple and you step outside into a new world of freedom. Notice how different your entire body and energy body feels now. You thank the temple and your wise being for your healing and with a lightness in your movement, you retrace your steps back to where you began.

You are now aware of your physical body, your breath, the sounds inside and outside the room. When you are ready, breathe in and open your eyes to the new you.

KEY LESSONS FROM CHAPTER FIFTEEN

- **We are part of a greater consciousness and a collective oneness**

- **To connect with your ever-present soul, practice stilling your mind**

- **Your greatness is bigger than you can ever imagine possible**

- **The possibilities of life are limitless and you can tune into whatever frequency you choose to experience**

CHAPTER SIXTEEN

Completing Your MindBody Journey

It's time to let go of the past that you are still carrying around with you, the past that keeps showing up in your body and in life and holding you back from creating the future you want to start living today.

We are not victims, we are creators. We create our lives from the inside out. Feeling joy and bliss is our natural state of being. Children still feel this. They see life very differently to us adults. Why? What stopped this happiness? Children fall and quickly pick themselves up and start to run again. When we have a fall in life, it seems to take us a lot longer to pick ourselves back up and start all over again!

What would it be like if you could feel your feelings then move on, without getting stuck in the feeling? It takes practice to stop holding on to life's dramas, to go with the flow, to allow and acknowledge your feelings, then move on. So it's time for you to stop getting stuck. Time to enjoy the mystery of life. Enjoy the process. Nothing is wrong. Judge less, listen more. As the inspirational author and mindfulness teacher Thich Nhat Hanh says, 'There is no way to happiness. Happiness is the way!'

Throughout Your MindBody Journey you have been uncovering your unconscious beliefs and the MindBody programming that has blocked you from having full health, happiness and fulfilment. This final exercise will help you to release this patterning and rewire your programming. This is a physical transformation that happens to your synapses in your brain.

The function of your synapses is to transfer electric activity (information) from one cell to another. The transfer can be from nerve to nerve (neuro-neuro), or nerve to muscle (neuro-myo). In other words you will literally be rewiring your brain, from old programming to new, which will change the information being sent to your body.

Your body and mind respond to ritual and repetition. For lasting change, you will need to consciously let go of old patterns of behaviour and keep on track maintaining your new habits. The key is consistence, persistence and patience. Remember once you have done this for a while, it will then become part of your new programming and your new habits will be absorbed into your unconscious and will then run on autopilot. Your work will then be done!

Shortly you will be performing a ritual. Rituals are very powerful, especially when the intention you bring to the ritual is strong. In ancient times ritual was part of daily life. Our ancestors understood the power of directed thought, intention and action. It was how the magic of manifestation happened. Today the true understanding of the power of ritual has been lost. However modern rituals which can include weddings, christenings, going to work at the same time, having our morning cup of tea or coffee, brushing our teeth are all making statements that we are serious and committed. Positive daily ritual is the act of taking positive thoughts and putting them into action. Once a positive ritual takes hold in your life, you don't even need to think about it. Just like brushing your teeth —it just happens.

This following ritual is a one off, but you will continue to feel the power of this ritual because you have set the intention. To keep the change process alive it is important you keep feeding your intention with a daily ritual that works best for you.

Are you ready to fully change your beliefs, reprogram your thoughts and transform your life? Are you ready to fully release your old, unconsciously programmed self and re-discover the real you?

Now it is time to write your final affirmation. Taking into account all you have discovered about yourself, all the old ways gone, all the new ways to embrace. You might want to use a combination of words from your previous affirmations you have written. With all this in mind (and body) write a new story, phrase or words for yourself that describes a new positive, powerful mindset for a new you.

My affirmation to reprogram my MindBody is:...............

....

....

This is your new MindBody mantra. Read it aloud with conviction as many times a day as you can and 'feel' the words when you speak them. Do this for the next few weeks or until you have embodied the phrase and it has become real and true for you. The more you say your affirmation with belief and conviction, the quicker it will become true. Your MindBody responds to ritual and repetition, so notice what shows up in your life as a result! Keep this affirmation by your bedside or carry it around with you to keep the new you energised.

You are now ready to walk into your new life.

A New Beginning Starts Now

Anything and everything is possible once your blocks of resistance have been removed. For example I would never have believed I could write a book. I believed I was stupid, the 'thicket' of the family (as my father affectionately used to call me not realising the negative programming he was setting up deep inside of me). My older sister was the brainy one and was encouraged to do well at school, which she did. I on the other hand was hopeless. My spelling was awful and I failed my English exam three times, being rated 'U' for 'ungraded'! I also had dyscalculia, which is a very hard word for me to spell and basically it means I was rubbish with numbers!

I seemed incapable of retaining the most basic information and spent most of my school life gazing out of the window! Art college seemed like the only place of higher education that would have me! So instead I focused on my artistic skills and with sheer determination to prove to everyone I was NOT a 'thicket', I worked my way up a career ladder in design, advertising and then publishing. By the age of 25, I had become the art editor for one of the UK's leading health magazines, which ironically lead me onto the healing path I am on now. Looking back, not only was I out to prove everyone wrong, but I also wanted to prove to myself that I was capable and I wanted to believe in myself. I wanted acceptance not just from others, but also from myself.

I realise now that I wasn't 'stupid' I just hadn't found anything interesting enough to hold my focus, I hadn't found my passion, and my purpose but for years I went around believing I was a hopeless failure and a 'thicket'. Only until I had changed my programming (and I did it the hard way, unconsciously) was I able to relate to myself as someone who was capable, even successful. I learnt to love myself, not for what I did, but for who I was. I could finally see beyond my pain, suffering and the illusions I had created for myself and woke up to who I truly am.

I love this quote by Marianne Williamson, from her book 'A Return To Love':

"Our deepest fear is not that we are inadequate. Our deepest fear is that we are powerful beyond measure. It is our light, not our darkness that most frightens us. We ask ourselves, 'Who am I to be brilliant, gorgeous,   talented, fabulous?' Actually, who are you not to be? You are a child of God. Your playing small does not serve the world. There is nothing enlightened about shrinking so that other people won't feel insecure around you. We are all meant to shine, as children do. We were born to make manifest the glory of God that is within us. It's not just in some of us; it's in everyone. And as we let our own light shine, we unconsciously give other people permission to do the same. As we are liberated from our own fear, our presence automatically liberates others."

Exercise #21:
Becoming The Person You Were Born To Be

It is best to read through this last exercise first as preparation is needed for your ritual and you might want to know what your ritual involves.

You will need a pen and two pieces of plain paper about A5 in size, you will also need either a match and a fire proof container, a dustbin that will be collected soon, or a flush lavatory! Pick one of these and have them handy. You will also need a mirror. A full length mirror is best, but a face mirror will do.

This final exercise is a very important, so make sure you honour this time and allow at least half an hour to spare where you won't be interrupted or disturbed.

Prepare yourself before you begin by washing your hands, going to the lavatory and turning off your electrical devices. Firstly on one piece of paper write the word 'OLD' on the back in big letters. Then on the other side of the piece of paper write any words of self talk that you have used that no longer serve you. They include all the negative words you have already written down from your exercises. Make sure you include the words or phrases you used for your 'story' in chapter 14.

They could also be words that describe ways you behave that you want to let got of. Take your time to get it all down, all the parts of yourself you have uncovered throughout your journey.

Now take the other piece of paper and write in big letters on one side the word 'NEW'. Turn the paper over and on the other side write words or a sentence of how you want to be in the future (remember your meditation at the end of chapter 10). Capture the words of how you might 'feel' as that new person. Or you might want to use your written affirmations from your exercises. You will use words or phrases to describe the person you want to be once all your pain, sufferings, grievances have been removed. Keep the words in the present moment. You might use words like this for example: I AM NOW happy, joyful, successful, passionate, confident, healthy, assertive, loving, compassionate, kind, abundant, wealthy, free etc.

Once you have finished writing all that you need to, put this piece of paper to the side for the moment.

Now you have two pieces of paper, one old and one new. Pick up your 'OLD' paper with your right hand and take another look at what you have written.

Get a sense of how the words make you feel. What do you feel in your body? Now know that the words you wrote do not describe the true you. At some point this belief about yourself was set up to protect you. Now we will take it a step further. Draw a line under your words and write underneath them any grievances or past hurts that you believe are still stuck within your energy system. What happened to you that took away your childlike innocence. What happened to you that took away your confidence, your love, your trust, your safety? What are you still carrying? Write any memories of your past that came up while reading this book. When you have written all you need to, look at your words. See how much you have been carrying. No wonder you don't have full health, full vitality, full happiness and joy. You don't deserve to carry this any longer.

I will now ask you an important question. Are you ready to let go of your past and let go of the 'OLD' you? You need to be sure. If you are not sure, that's OK, just give yourself time to consider your reasons why. Why do you want to hold on to the old you? What are you afraid of losing? Giving up? Facing? When all the resistance to letting go of the old has gone, place your 'OLD' words in your right hand and take a look at yourself in a mirror. It is best to view your whole body if you can. Look at your body and notice how much it has been carrying for you over the years. Notice where the load is the most? Notice where the strain has been the greatest. Look at your face, see how your expression has adopted all the words you have written on your paper. Look into your eyes and notice all the pain and suffering you have ever felt that has taken away your sparkle.

It is time to call your spirit back, the true you before you were controlled by your fears, mind and emotions, before your defence mechanisms were set up. It's time to reclaim your true self and bring back your soul fragments that were lost along your way. It's time to call your true spirit back to become the person you were born to be.

Thank the old you for all it has done to serve you so far, you acknowledge it has been there to serve and protect you, but you kindly tell the old you it is now time to go. Say 'thank you' and now take a deep breath in and declare out loud, 'I now release my old patterning'. Say this out loud three times and with an out breath, either tear up your paper, into tiny pieces, set fire to it safely or if you think it's appropriate, flush it down the toilet. Make sure the paper has fully gone, by either putting the ashes or torn up paper in an outside bin, or taking it to a public trash bin. You have now fully left the old behind. Notice in your body how that feels.

Now pick up your 'NEW' paper in your left hand and look at your words again and get a sense of how the words make you feel. Where do you feel the words in your body? This is you, the real you with all your fears removed. This is your true spirit before all your heartbreaks, your disillusions, your suffering and pain. It's time to come back home to you. Keep reading your words and allow the feelings behind your words to expand. Welcome these words, become these feelings, acknowledge that this is who you truly are when your resistance and blocks are removed. This is you now and in your future. Again look at yourself in the mirror. Look at your eyes, see deep into your eyes and see the little child that you once were, wide-eyed with wonder, sparkling with innocence and joy, excited about your life ahead.

See yourself as you truly are, see through to the depths of your soul. Feel the love in your eyes from your soul pouring out towards you. Say hello and welcome in the new you.

Now lay or sit in a comfortable position and place your 'NEW' paper on the part of your body that you had the most issues, physically or emotionally. Once you have read the below, close your eyes and do your final meditation.

Allow the words on your 'NEW' paper to penetrate your body. Feel it in every nerve, cell, muscle, fibre of your being. Tune in to your heart centre and feel a warm loving glow, all is well and you are loved deeply. Imagine a white light of pure love radiating from your heart and to your entire being.

You are back to the pure beautiful you that you have always been. Your limitations have been stripped away, your programming has been dissolved. The new you has been born.

You can tune into this feeling anytime you wish as it is now a part of you. It is the real you. Stay in this place of love, peace and happiness for as long as you feel you need to, the when you are ready, open your eyes.

Again face the mirror and see your body as the new you. Notice how different you look. Not only do you have a new body, but you have new eyes to see your body freshly. Has your posture changed? Has your face changed? Has your attitude changed? Look deep into your eyes, is there anything different? What do you notice?

It's your turn now, to see and believe in who you really are. You are an awesome vibrant light and it shines wherever you go. You are love in action and that love constantly touches others. This beautiful planet you live on is a magical playground full of possibilities and you were put on it for a reason. You are a vital part of the evolutionary process. You are special and unique like no-one else on this planet. You are brave enough to follow your heart and not your fears. You are wise enough to listen to your inner guidance to fulfil your inner most dreams.

And when you do this, you allow others to do so too, helping the world to vibrate in perfect harmony.

Anything is possible for you now, all you need to do is believe.

30 Top Tips to keep you on track with your new life:

1. Repeat your MindBody Mantra as often as you can.
2. Change your daily routines to break your bad habits.
3. Live in the moment as opposed to the future or past.
4. Whenever a fear-based thought arises, replace it with love-based thoughts.
5. Move your body regularly in the form of exercise, this will help to replenish your cells with oxygen which is vital for your body to work efficiently.
6. Respect your body by eating healthily.
7. Pause and feel the magic in every moment.
8. Put your dreams into action.
9. Focus on what's right and not what's wrong.
10. Judge less, listen more.
11. Get out of your head and into your heart.
12. Be authentic and honest.
13. Feel gratitude and look for things to be grateful for.
14. Let go of toxic relationships.
15. Stop yourself when you hear a negative thought and change it to a positive one.
16. Express your emotions then move on.
17. Give thanks for all you do have, as opposed to focussing on what you don't have.
18. Laugh more, sing more, dance more.
19. Use the word 'love' more in your vocabulary.
20. Hug people from your heart.
21. Be compassionate, but stay emotionally detached from other people's problems.
22. Take responsibility for your own health, happiness, and life and don't blame others.
23. Spend more time in nature to keep yourself in touch with whats real.
24. Forgive your past and look forward to your future.
25. Breathe deeply (often).
26. Listen to your body and the messages it gives you.
27. Love the beautiful person that you are!
28. Surround yourself with people that nourish you.
29. Don't just do what you love, learn to love what you do.
30. Be happy!

If you would like me to keep you posted, here is a list of useful links:

- If you would like to share your stories about what you discovered on Your MindBody Journey, I'd love to hear from you. Email me at: **jakkie@mindbodycourses.com**

- If you would like to become a member of my MindBody mailing list to keep you posted with more tips and tools then sign up at: **www.mindbodycourses.com/loginjoin-page**

- To help you on your new journey, personal Affirmation products are available by me through: **www.artbyjakkie.weebly.com www.zazzle.com.au/artandsoulbyjakkie**

- If you would like to see if there's a workshop near you visit: **www.mindbodycourses.com/courses-available**

- If you would like me to hold a workshop in your area contact me on: **jakkie@mindbodycourses.com**

- If you would like a one-to-one **MindBody consultation** or **coaching session** with me on either Skype, FaceTime, Messenger, Viber, WhatsApp or Google Hangouts, please get in touch to book an appointment.

ACKNOWLEDGMENTS

Thank you to all my beloved clients over the many years for being such special spirits, who have been brave enough to open your hearts, minds and souls and for sharing the scary stuff with me. I honour and admire you all!!

A huge thank you to my dear family for putting up with my free spirit and my crazy ideas. I am so sorry for breaking your hearts every time I decide to live on the other side of the world to you.

Thank you Andria my best friend in the whole wide world for getting me, loving me unconditionally and supporting me on my life's journey. Holding hands forever baaaaaaaaaby!

Also big hug for my soul sister Helen for your endless belief and encouragement.

Big thanks to my Aussie family Ian, Natalie and Jayden for all your support over our many shared years Down Under. I feel so grateful to all my friends for touching my heart and being at the right place at the right time to share the special moments with.

Finally, a special thank you to my partner Glen Poole for helping me shape my ideas and share them with the world. You are a master in your own right and I am so proud of all you do for the world, particularly in your life's work for men and boys. Not only are you the love of my life but also my inspiration and my mentor. I appreciate all our shared laughs, our tears and our crazy dancing!

I love you all   x

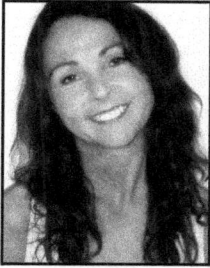

ABOUT THE AUTHOR

Jakkie Talmage is a writer, artist, therapist, healer, teacher, spiritual coach and the founder of the MindBody Courses UK.

Formally the art editor for one of the UK's leading complimentary health magazine's, she was inspired to unplug from corporate life and pursue a more natural lifestyle. After a year travelling the world, Jakkie emigrated to Australia and created a new life for herself.

Jakkie is passionate about helping people discover their own healing, their inner wisdom and their personal power and has helped hundreds of people in the UK and Australia.

In meditation, she was guided to put her existing 12 week course 'The MindBody Journey' into this book to reach a wider audience, as she believes everyone has the right to remember their ancient wisdom and to have tools to enable them to live the life intended for them. This is one of health, happiness, success and inner peace.

To help support people on their journey of transformation, Jakkie has created a range of affirmation products. Art & Soul designs are colourful images with inspirational words on everyday products which uplift and inspire.

Jakkie communes with nature everyday, as this is where she gets her inspiration and connects to spirit. She currently lives in Australia with her partner and continues to run workshops, seminars, retreats and one-to-one consultations in Australia and the UK.

REFERENCES

Heal your body - Louise Hay

Bodymind - Ken Dychwald

Somatics - Thomas Hanna

The power of focussing - Ann Weiser Cornell

Your body believes every word you say -

Barbara Hoberman Levine

The mindbody prescription - John E Sarno MD

The biology of belief - Bruce lipton

How your mind can heal your body -

David R Hamilton PHD

What everybody is saying - Joe Navarro

The bodymind workbook - Debbie Shapiro

The body is the barometer of the soul - Annette Noontil

Conscious medicine - Gill Edwards

Anatomy of the spirit - Caroline Myss PHD

The hidden messages in water - Masaru Emoto